D1272948

A Manual Of Hospital Podiatry

By

PATRICK A. DeMOON, Executive Director
Franklin Boulevard Community Hospital —
Central Community Hospital
Lecturer in Hospital Protocol
Illinois College of Podiatric Medicine
Founder of the National Academy of Hospital Podiatry

and

O. A. MERCADO, D.P.M.
Chairman, Department of Surgery,
Illinois College of Podiatric Medicine
Chairman, Department of Podiatry,
Franklin Boulevard Community Hospital

Published By
THE NATIONAL ACADEMY OF HOSPITAL PODIATRY
Franklin Boulevard Community Hospital
3240 West Franklin Boulevard
Chicago, Illinois 60624

TABLE OF CONTENTS

FOREWORD

As early as 1925 Podiatric Surgery was taught to the students of the Illinois College of Podiatric Medicine and its affiliate the Chicago Foot Clinics. A limited number of podiatrists were performing surgical procedures in their offices. Hospital podiatry surgery was non-existent at that time.

In the late 40's and early 50's a small number of podiatrists were given limited privileges at a few scattered medical and osteopathic hospitals. These privileges were for inpatient or outpatient services with no formal guidelines developed for the hospital affiliations.

By 1960, and especially with the inclusion of the guidelines for podiatric surgical services by the Joint Commission on Accreditation of Hospitals, a number of podiatrists were accepted as members of the hospital podiatric surgical staff.

At the present time hundreds of Medical and Osteopathic hospitals in the United States have opened up their surgical departments to qualified podiatrists.

For those members of the podiatry profession who are qualified to perform surgical procedures and do not as yet have hospital privileges, this book is invaluable. Entering a hospital complex is akin to taking up residency in a foreign country. Everything is strange and the organizational activities are sometimes beyond comprehension.

It is most important for the doctor who seeks to obtain hospital privileges to have a complete and thorough understanding and appreciation for all hospital organizations and activities. He must learn how he will function best on the hospital team. This "Manual of Hospital Podiatry" by Patrick A. DeMoon and O. A. Mercado, D.P.M., will do much to bridge the gap that exists between office and hospital podiatry practice.

In conclusion, it must always be understood that the hospital exists primarily for the good and welfare of the patient. Every activity, every service and every individual working in a hospital must carry out his or her functions in the best interests of the patient and that includes the chief of the surgical staff as well as the orderly on the floor.

While a reading of this manual offers no guarantee that it will get you a hospital appointment, it will bring you one step closer to that goal.

Phillip R. Brachman, D.P.M., President
Illinois College of Podiatric Medicine

A History of Podiatry

Many members of the general public see the profession of podiatry as a young field in the healing arts, few realize how far back in time the art and science of podiatry really goes. Actually, the first case is pictured as long ago as 372 B.C. when the Greek Theophrastus talked about bunions and their cure and Hikesios in Smyrna (in 60 A.D.) prepared special plasters for their treatment.

In Northern Europe in the 14th century, the Guild of Barber-Surgeons provided such services as pulling teeth, cutting corns, trimming nails, bloodletting, applying leeches and compounding formulas for the relief of pain. You might say that these barber-surgeons were the forerunners of today's surgery, dentistry, and podiatry. Of course, medicine and dentistry eventually came into their own as vital and respected professions while podiatry more slowly developed into a separate division of the healing art.

Today, foot care comes under the general term of podiatry. Originally, however, it was known as "chiropody", having been so designated by David Low, an Englishman, in 1784. He adapted it from the French word "chirurgien" (surgeon) and pied (foot) or literally, "surgeon of the foot."

If one goes back to the late 1800's, he will find that the calling of chiropody fell to anyone who desired to engage in it, including many door-to-door traveling corn cutters, who came with their tools in a bag to solicit business.

Podiatry in America really got under way during the early part of the nineteenth century when a few people with some basic knowledge of their craft began to offer their services to people troubled by foot ailments. The art they practiced was brought to America from Europe, where the Guild of Barber-Surgeons mentioned previously treated the foot ailments of the nobility, royalty and the rich.

In 1846, an itinerant corn cutter named Nehemia Kenison was making a fair living treating the feet of New England mill workers. Finally, in that same year, he opened an office in Boston which dealt solely with foot care. From this early beginning has emerged a highly specialized profession dedicated and devoted to caring for the human foot.

Perhaps the most recent official offshoot of the medical profession, present-day podiatry boasts some 8,800 members in the United States, the majority of whom operate in the larger population centers. Today, podiatrists are in offices, although six or seven percent now practice their profession in hospitals and nursing homes.

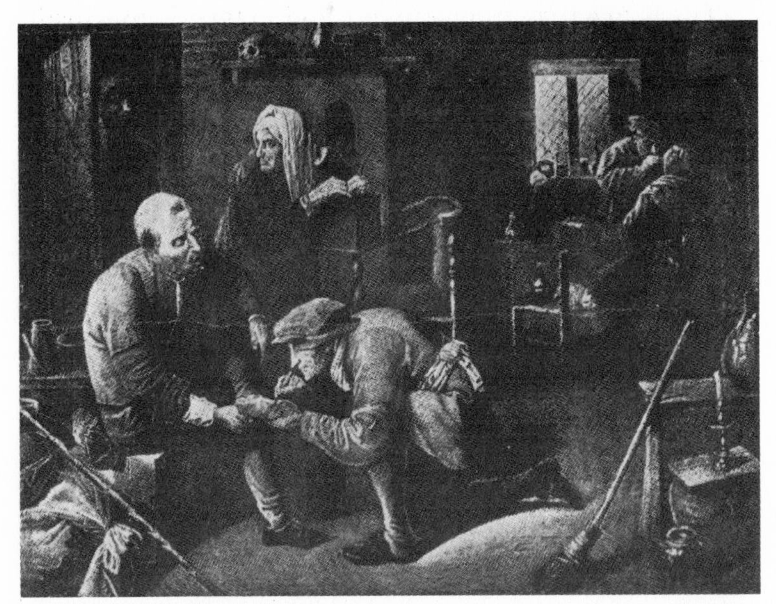

This is the old-fashioned chiropodist or corn cutter, who often traveled door to door, practicing his rather primitive craft.

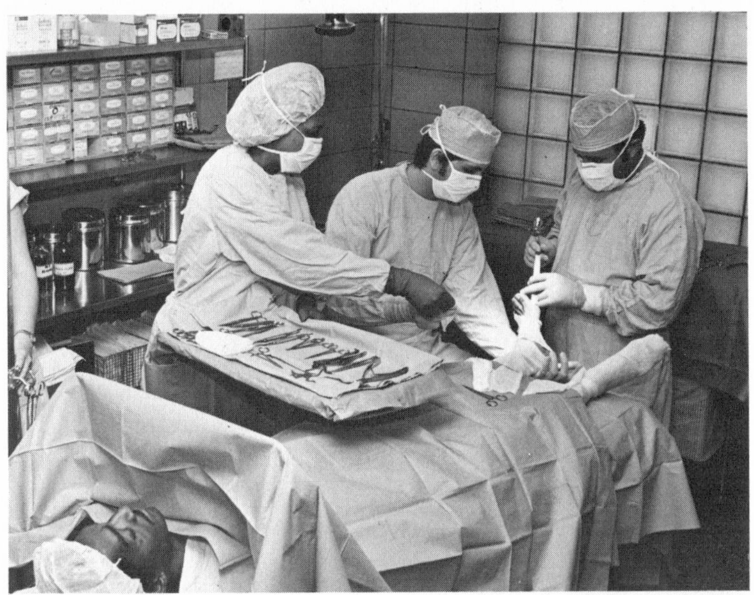

Today's modern, podiatric surgeon performing his highly technical surgical operations is a far cry indeed from the early practitioners of the profession.

There are five, independently-chartered, non-profit colleges of podiatric medicine in the United States, the first of which was opened in 1911. They enroll about 1,800 students and annually graduate about 250 D.P.M.'s. In the beginning, these schools were developed by podiatrists with little help from outside sources. However, today these colleges receive federal grants for construction of physical facilities and for carrying on their programs of education. Some states also financially support the podiatry colleges within their borders.

Of the 275 teachers who staff the five colleges, about 150 are podiatrists. The others are doctors of medicine and philosophy and more of these are coming in as the horizons of podiatry are enlarged and expanded.

In the United States, as we have mentioned, the battle to be properly recognized and respected was begun by podiatrists at about the beginning of the century. Perhaps a reason for the lack of progress through the years is so few advances made in the science of podiatry during this early period. Podiatrists did their business in a traditional, plodding and unimaginative manner and while they were respectable people, they themselves were not respected. When podiatric development began to surge forward, with new discoveries, better methods of operating, more knowledgeable results, podiatry gradually began to come into its own.

The modern, college-trained podiatrist who has kept up with the advancing times and who performs his tasks with judgement, technical skill and competence, can be on a par with any other physician. He will make an excellent living, win honors as a health professional and his judgements will be respected.

Podiatry and the Health Team

There has been much discussion regarding the most effective way to combine individual medical practices and huge health-care systems. An important segment of this picture is evaluating the educational requirements, responsibility and relationship between physicians, practitioners of specialties and technicians working in the health field. If you can forget the early, unhappy image of the practicing podiatrist, you will see in today's modern, up-to-date practitioner a man of extensive technical skills. But there are still numerous physicians who do not consider podiatrists the appropriate Referral for their patient's foot problems. In many cases, they are older men, and their memories of the chiropodist type of podiatry practitioner gives them no reassurance. They feel that podiatrists are competent to do only palliative corn, callus and toenail care. But how competently can the podiatrist approach a diabetic ulcer? Would he know when to refer a foot edema to the physician as a possible cause of heart failure? Dr. Richard N. Podell cites one orthopedic surgeon who said, "Podiatrists are not trained to and do not recognize the systemic implications of what they see on the foot. Only a physician can do this. Let's face it, there is no such thing as a half-doctor."

The real trouble is that the physician who criticizes the podiatrist has little firm knowledge of or experience with modern podiatry education and practice. Certainly there are some podiatrists who would not recognize the systemic implications of some conditions but those who have kept up or who have had current training in good schools, in modern, medically-oriented curriculums, are definitely capable of this knowledge.

Podiatry has come a long way from the early days. Specialization has brought a vast new knowledge and experience of the craft and fine techniques have been developed which make competent craftsmanship infinitely easier. In addition, to quote a dedicated podiatrist. "For most surgeons and orthopedists, the foot is not an exciting organ. Podiatrists give the foot greater tender loving care. After all, it's all we've got"!

If we are to be realistic, then we can say that podiatric students should definitely be trained to recognize the systemic implications of foot disease and refer such cases to physicians for corroborative diagnosis and systemic therapy. Knowledge is never wasted, it is the bloom on the rose, it is the extra asset that can introduce the podiatrist to the aura of professional respectability with the physician and a permanent and happy place in the hospital scene.

The Education of the Podiatrist

There are five accredited podiatry colleges in America. It is not generally known but the legal minimum undergraduate requirements for podiatry colleges are virtually identical to those of medical school. Indeed in the modern podiatric college, the curriculum is surprisingly similar to that of the medical school. The first two years are devoted largely to general anatomy, biochemistry, physiology, embryology, bacteriology, pathology, and pharmacology. Students learn the histology of the myocardium and the effects of digitalis as well as the vasculature of the foot.

Most podiatric colleges spend most of their second, third, and fourth years in supervised patient care.

There are, in addition, seminars and workshops on general medicine, anesthesia, peripheral vascular disease, diabetes, general surgery, physical medicine, orthopedics and community podiatry. Students who are taught physical diagnosis in the medical wards are asked to recognize mitral rumbles and to note increased jugular pressure.

Formal, post-doctoral training for podiatrists is not required in many states but a considerable group of podiatry graduates have commenced serving formal internships and even residencies. In this country today, there are 111 one year-long hospital-based podiatry internships and 50 more are in the planning stage. Each year marks the graduation of approximately 250 Doctors of Podiatric Medicine (D.P.M.) to swell the ranks of the profession.

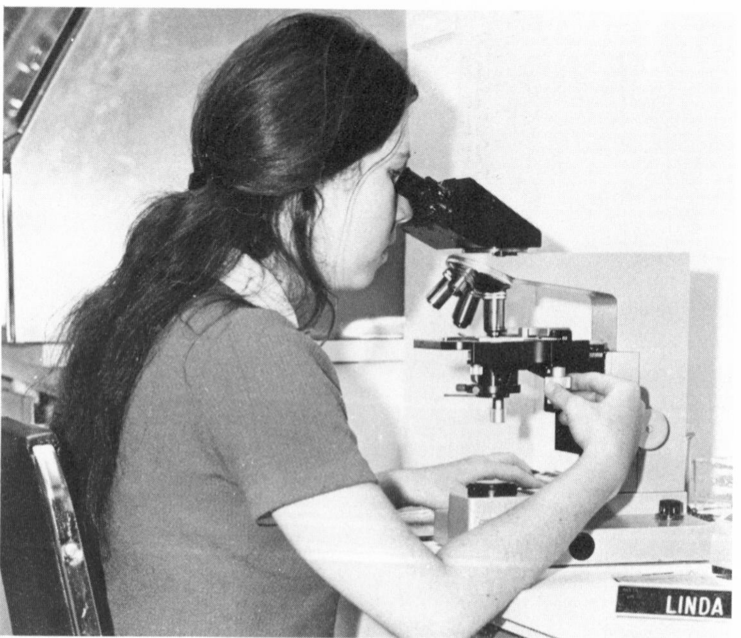

Biochemistry and physiology, embryology, bacteriology and pathology are an important part of the podiatrist's curriculum.

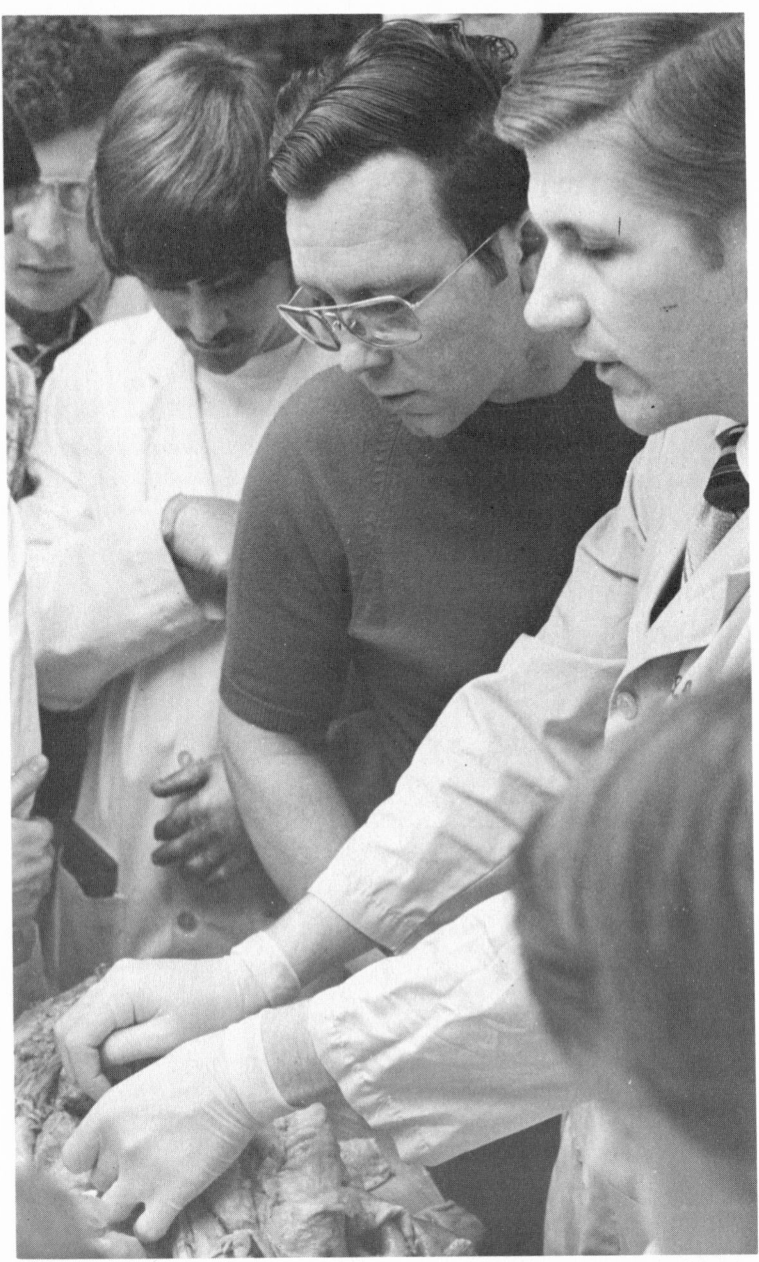

The curriculum in today's modern podiatric college is surprisingly similar to that of any accredited medical school. Here an anatomy lecture is being given to several students.

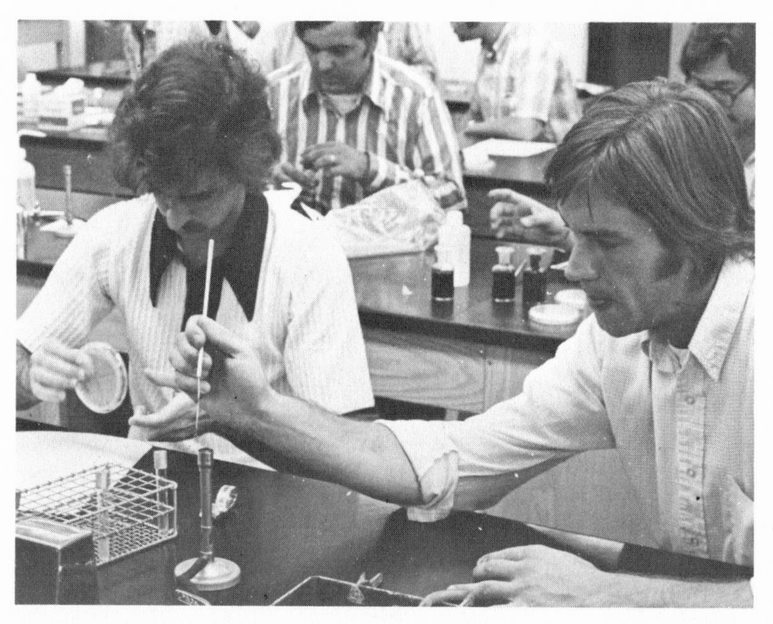

Students spend a good portion of their first two years at school in laboratory studies.

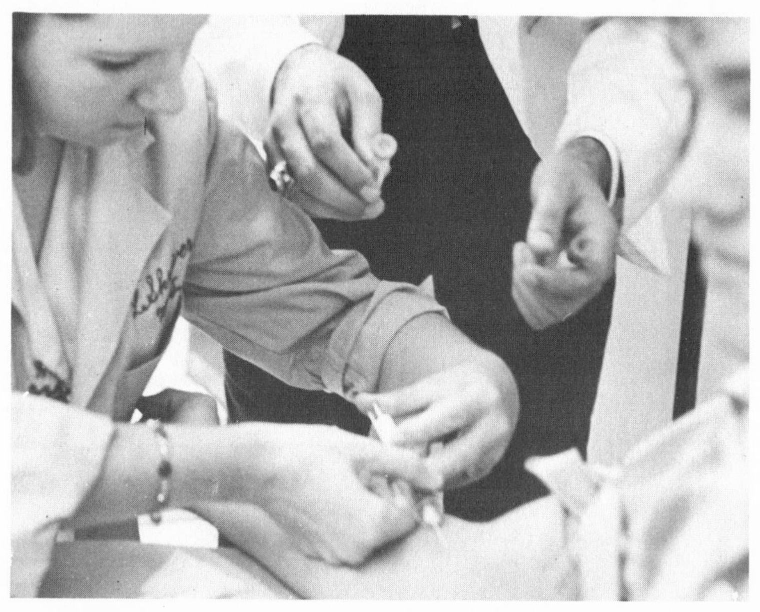

Under supervision of competent instructors and practitioners, students learn the latest in medical techniques.

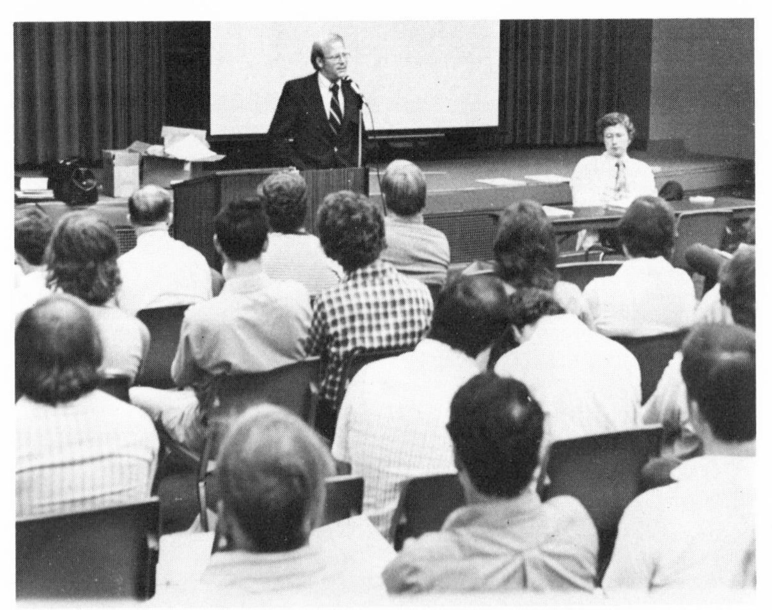

The didactic material given in classes is reinforced by practical applications in the clinics.

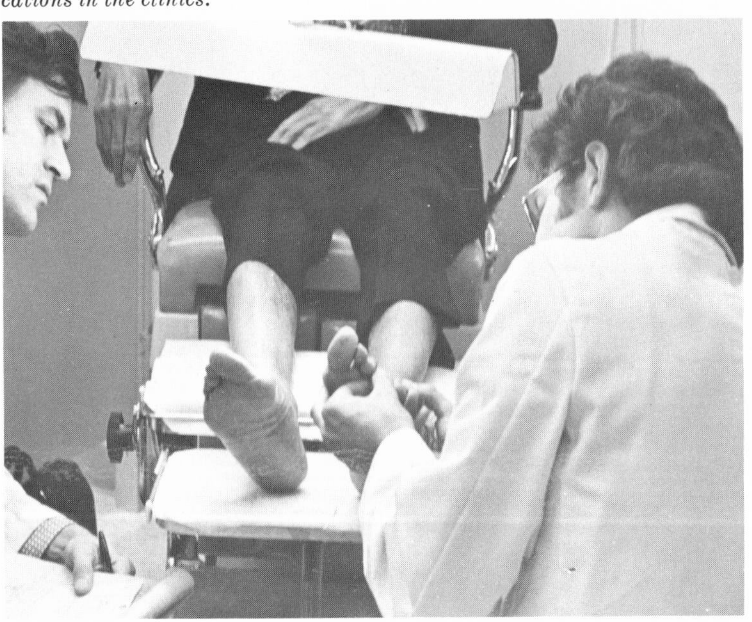

History taking and physical diagnosis are a big part of the college routine.

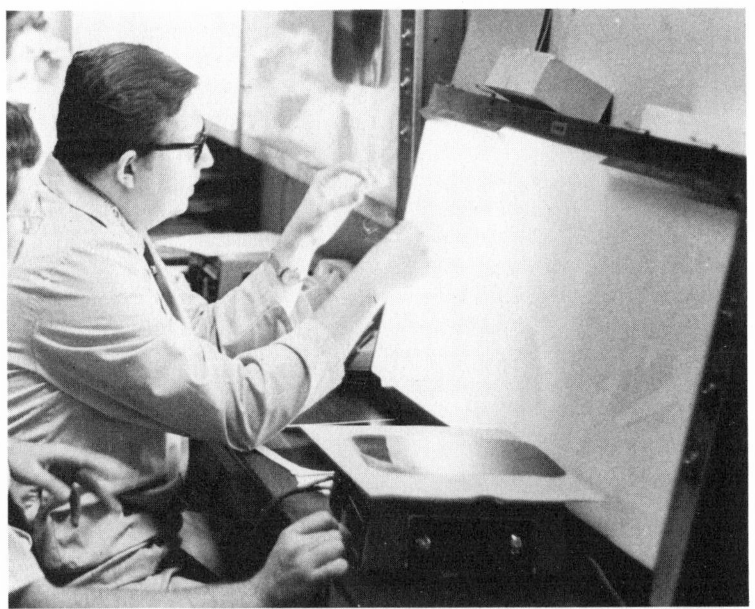

X-rays are an important part of the podiatrist's practice and reading them is an art to be learned from experienced practitioners.

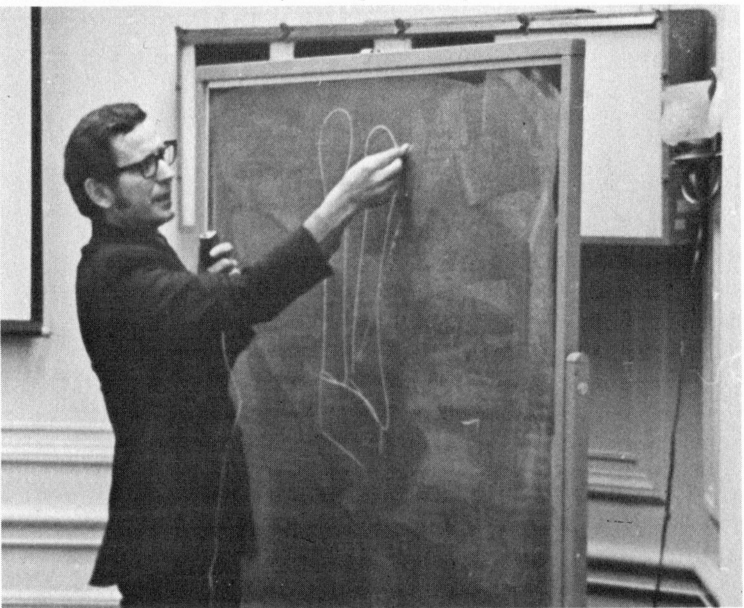

Lectures by prominent podiatric surgeons is an essential part of training the student.

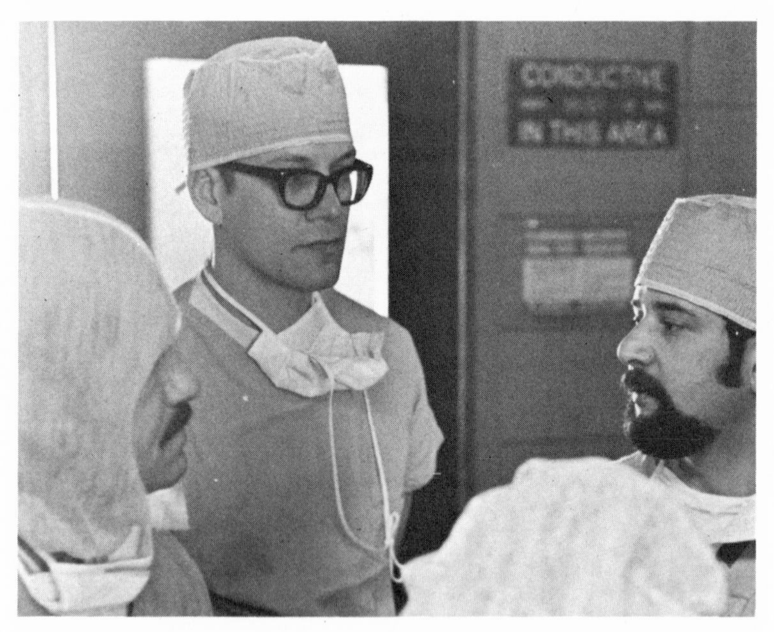

A podiatric surgeon explains a surgical technique to his students.

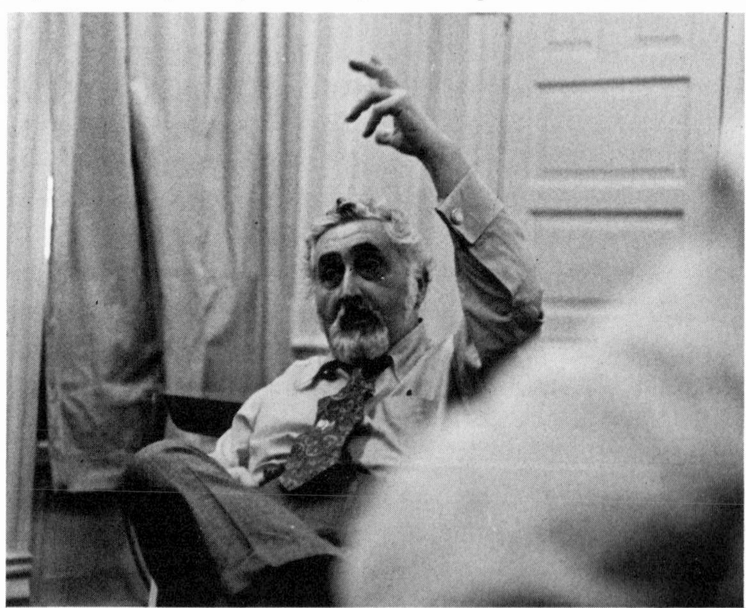

A distinguished internist-teacher lectures a group of podiatric students on some of the intricacies of internal medicine.

The Practice of Podiatry

Podiatry is no longer a small-time operation. The number of people visiting podiatrists yearly run into the millions. Many additional millions suffer from foot problems. Yet it is amazing what a small percentage of Americans have real understanding of the podiatrist and what he does. The situation literally cries for creative and constructive public relations to make both the physicians and the masses aware of the burgeoning aspects of this profession, its potential for doing good, its willingness to provide care, and more than all these, the comfort it can bring to the huge army which suffers from foot ailments.

Over 8000 podiatrists are currently practicing their craft in this country. The laws vary from state to state but in many of these, podiatry is defined as "The diagnosis, medical, physical, or surgical treatment of ailments of the human foot, with the exception of administration of general anesthetics, or amputation of the foot." In a number of states the law also includes the treatment of the leg. The podiatrist is able to prescribe drugs for disease and control of pain, including narcotics.

If one should examine the national picture regarding the distribution of podiatrists, he would find that nationally, the ratio is approximately 4.1 podiatrists per 100,000 persons. In the Eastern states, there are 7.2 podiatrists per 100,000 and in the Southern states, only 1.9.

As is known, the greater number of podiatrists in this country are in private practice, the majority of them in general practice. Many of the younger podiatrists, the newer graduates, however, have qualified to practice such specialties as foot orthopedics, foot surgery, foot roentgenology, or podiatric dermatology. Curiously, more than 95% of our practicing podiatrists are male and 95% are white.

About 50% of the patients who visit a podiatrist have only the average corn-callus-toenail problems. But there are many other ills, some of them quite serious, with important systemic manifestations. To quote a few examples: diabetic ulcers, fungal infections, cellulitis, manifestations of sickle cell disease, gout, rheumatoid arthritis, osteoarthritis, flatfoot, leg, hip, and spinal deformities, neoplasm, psychiatric disease, venous incompetence, and the edema of right-side heart failure. So, one can understand, the podiatrist is being called upon to function in an ever-widening range of medical specialties.

Richard N. Podell, M.D., distinguished physician and author and the source of many of these facts, estimates that one-fifth of all podiatry visits involve surgical procedures, about 10% of them having to do with surgery on the bone, muscle, tendon or joint. "Probably the most frequent orthopedic surgical procedures in podiatry", says Dr. Podell, "are the correction of 'Hammer toes', to prevent recurrence of corns, and repair of bunions (hallux valgus). The former is often an office procedure, the latter is usually done in a hospital. More complicated orthopedic surgery such as reconstructive surgery or arthrodesis was not done by podiatrists until a very few years ago." Since the advent of hospital affiliations, however, operations of this nature are beginning to be performed more frequently.

There is no question that, if modern podiatry is to be practiced effectively, access to hospitals or the existence of a podiatric section in hospitals is essential. The Joint Commission on the Accreditation of Hospitals has given the individual hospital the right to decide whether podiatrists should have admitting privileges. A member of the hospital's medical staff must co-sponsor each admission and assume responsibility for the patient's over-all care. Although, a small number of hospitals around the country grant podiatrists in-patient privileges, the list is growing and we will see the day when podiatry will have sections in every major hospital in the nation.

The Joint Commission Rules on Podiatrists in the Hospital

The successful emergence of the podiatrists in the American hospital scene was made possible through Bulletin 44 of the Joint Commission on Accreditation of Hospitals, published in 1967. This Bulletin and the Joint Commission's new and enlightened stand on podiatry was principally brought about through the efforts of Douglas T. Mowbray, D.P.M., representing the podiatric profession and John D. Porterfield, M.D., Director, Joint Commission on Accreditation of Hospitals.

Most interesting are the words of the Commission on this special subject, reading as follows:

"The governing body of the hospital, after considering the recommendations of a medical staff, may grant clinical privileges to qualified, licensed podiatrists in accordance with their training, experience and demonstrated competence and judgment. When this is done, podiatrists must comply with all applicable medical staff bylaws, rules and regulations, which must contain specific references governing podiatric services.

"A podiatrist with clinical privileges may, with the concurrence of an appropriate member of the medical staff, initiate the procedure for admitting a patient. This concurring medical staff member shall assume responsibility for the overall aspects of the patient's care throughout the hospital stay, including the medical history and physical examination. Patients admitted to the hospital for podiatric care must be given the same basic medical appraisal as patients admitted for other services.

"The scope and extent of surgical procedures that each podiatrist may perform must be specifically defined and recommended in the same manner as all other surgical privileges. Surgical procedures performed by podiatrists must be under the overall supervision of the chief of surgery. The nature and degree of supervision is a matter of determination, in each instance, within the medical staff policy that governs the relationship and dual responsibility existing between the medical staff and the podiatrist. A physician member of the medical staff must be responsible for the care of any medical problem that may be present or that may arise during the hospitalization of podiatric patients. The podiatrist is responsible for the podiatric care of the patient, including the podiatric history and all appropriate elements of the patient's record. The podiatrist may write orders within the scope of his license, as limited by the applicable statutes and as consistent with the medical staff regulations."

On April 14, 1973, the Joint Commission made a number of changes to further clarify its stand on podiatry in the hospitals. These changes were duly noted in the Annual Report of the American Podiatry Association and read as follows:

1. The section on "Survey Eligibility Criteria" has been revised to clarify:
   a. that hospital admissions must be by a member of the medical staff "either individually or in cooperation with a podiatrist with clinical privileges."
   b. Only "licensed practitioners" (M.D., D.O., dentist and podiatrist) shall be directly responsible for diagnosis and treatment of patients.
   c. Other direct medical care to patients may be provided only by members of the "house staff" and by "other specified professional personnel."
2. The glossary definition of "house staff" has been expanded to include licensed practitioners, as well as graduates of medical, dental and podiatric schools in training programs approved by a nationally recognized accrediting agency, or established pursuant to state law. Such graduates may participate in patient care under the direction of licensed practitioners who have clinical privileges in the hospital.
3. A new glossary definition for "specified professional personnel" has been added. This category includes licensed practitioners, house staff, and "other personnel qualified to render direct medical care" under supervision of a practitioner

with clinical privileges. Such "other personnel" expressly refers to, among others, "medical, dental or podiatric students . . . who are participating in an intra-hospital educational clinical experience leading to graduation and/or qualification to state license examinations."

Concurrently, with the above changes, the Joint Commission also revised its Hospital Survey Questionnaire which the hospital administrator completes when the hospital is evaluated. The hospital must now certify that medical practice "is limited to appropriately licensed practitioners who have been granted clinical privileges within the limits of their qualifications" and that "clinical duties and responsibilities for segments of patient care are assigned to specified professional personnel."

In our view, the various statements of the Joint Commission referred to above, significantly clarify the status of a podiatrist to whom clinical privileges have been granted at a hospital. In addition, the role of podiatric residents and externs in approved training programs is recognized on a basis essentially equivalent to comparable medical and dental personnel.

Setting Up the Hospital Podiatry Section

Undoubtedly, the biggest problem the podiatrist has to face in advancing his career, is to approach a receptive hospital and persuade them to establish a Department of Podiatry. It is important that he not be disturbed by this chore, since more and more hospitals are consistently being made favorably aware of the importance of a hospital podiatry department within their walls.

We all know that a certain amount of politics is involved in what we are trying to do, so it is vital that a well-planned, quietly-positive attitude be taken in this matter rather than a negative one. Good public relations can be of inestimable help in one's quest.

There are many "pluses" on the side of the podiatrist seeking a hospital affiliation which we would like to discuss. For example, it is a fact that:

1. A Department of Podiatry in a hospital is a distinct asset, helping to improve patient care, which should always be the hospital's challenge and responsibility to the consuming public.
2. Hospitals throughout the nation which do have such departments, have learned that podiatric patients usually have short hospital stays and utilize all the hospital's profit-making departments—X-ray, Laboratory, etc. Little nursing care is required since they are not usually seriously ill and have an opportunity to enjoy the modern hospital's cuisine and services. Too, they often turn out to be the hospital's best public relations men!
3. Podiatric surgery is covered by all major insurance carriers, Medicare, and, in many states, Medicaid (welfare).
4. The podiatric patient is usually a working man or woman who has good insurance coverage and can pay his way in any hospital he visits.
5. Medical men who are concerned about the practice of podiatry in a hospital may be set at ease by the knowledge that this practice is limited to and consistent with the principles of the practice of podiatry established and recognized by the laws of their particular state.
6. The changes in the by-laws which are necessary for the inclusion of podiatry in a hospital service are minimal and most worthwhile. Since podiatry has already been given the blessing of the Joint Commission, it often requires only the mere agreement of the Medical Staff and the Board of Trustees to include a Department of Podiatry.

7. In these changing times, where the inevitability of socialized medicine must be accepted, podiatry continues to be a necessary medical discipline which should be included in every hospital.
8. Regarding the actual practice of podiatry in the Surgical Room (where there is the most opposition), it has been determined that once the podiatry department has been established, it functions well and becomes an integral part of the regular hospital service.
9. In the case of the Operating Room Supervisor, very little change is required from her normal OR techniques and only a handful of special instruments need be ordered. From the standpoint of surgical time, the podiatrist's cases are usually booked days and weeks ahead of time and many of the cases are of brief duration.

SURGICAL PRIVILEGES FOR PODIATRISTS

Podiatry is the only surgical specialty in medicine that has no Certificate Boards. We could editorialize a great deal on this subject but suffice to say that it is this lack of Board Certification which sometimes creates the biggest problem in the operating room. In hospitals throughout the country, regardless of their size, every man who enters the operating room must have a Surgical Control Card, which tells the Operating Room Supervisor which surgeries he is permitted to do and which he is not. Obviously, if a man is Board Certified such as, let us say, an orthopedic surgeon, there is no problem about qualifying him, since he has been qualified by his training and residency.

In similar manner, podiatric surgeons will eventually be certified throughout the country. There are dozens of residency programs now graduating top-notch podiatric surgeons who in future will insist upon being Board Certified.

But what do we do for the present? Obviously, the granting of surgical privileges to any podiatrist has to be through a peer mechanism. In other words, it is essential that the qualified podiatric surgeon be allowed to operate to the fullest extent of the law of the state and that he and the other qualified podiatrists on the staff be the "watch dogs" of this precious surgical privilege.

We feel strongly that surgical privileges should not be granted promiscuously but given in a graded and well-formulated manner according to the talents and proven abilities of the podiatrist.

The overseeing podiatrist, or Chief of the Podiatric Service, has a legal, as well as a moral, responsibility to the patient and the hospital to see that surgeons operating in his department are fully qualified to perform these operations and not attempting cases above their abilities or experience, since that could only bring disaster to the department.

The Control Card (reproduced below) is utilized at a number of hospitals throughout the country. This card does not limit the practice of podiatry, since the qualified surgeon who has full privileges, is permitted to perform any and all procedures in podiatry.

It is important that the podiatric surgeon designated to review surgical privileges be objective and fair but in no sense lenient in his decisions. His task is to make sure that the man performing the surgery has been fully qualified through a peer mechanism.

(front of card)

Name Office Address Phone

PODIATRIST ______________________________

has been assigned the following medical staff classification: ______________________

and may perform podiatry procedure as herewith indicated: ______________________

1 NAIL SURGERY

- ☐ Winograd Technique
- ☐ Frost Technique
- ☐ Terminal Syme Technique
- ☐ Kaplan Technique
- ☐ Verruca Resection Technique
- ☐ Verruca Needling Technique

2 DIGITAL SURGERY

- ☐ Heloma Durom
- ☐ Heloma Molle
- ☐ Hammer Toe
- ☐ Interactable Plantar Keratosis (soft tissue only)
- ☐ Bursectomy
- ☐ Neoplasm
- ☐ Mallet Toe
- ☐ Webbed Toes

3 NEOPLASM & FOREIGN OBJECTS

- ☐ Neuroma
- ☐ Foreign Body

METATARSAL SURGERY

- ☐ Hallux Rigidus
- ☐ Partial Metatarsal Head Resection
- ☐ Complete Metatarsal Head Resection
- ☐ Duvries Plantar Condylectomy
- ☐ Tailor's Bunion
- ☐ Freiberg's Infraction
- ☐ Hypertrophic Fifth Metatarsal Base

TENDON - LIGAMENT SURGERY

- ☐ Spring Ligament Shortening
- ☐ Tenotomy
- ☐ Tenectomy
- ☐ Ankle Ligament Stabilization
- ☐ Z-plasty
- ☐ Transplant

ACCESSORY BONE SURGERY

- ☐ Sesamoidectomy
- ☐ Osperoneum
- ☐ Os Vesalianum

(back of card)

4 MID-TARSAL SURGERY

- ☐ Navicular Ostectomy
- ☐ Calcaneal - Cuboidal Bridge
- ☐ Ostectomy Hyperostosis of Cuneiforms

HEEL SURGERY

- ☐ Haglunds Deformity
- ☐ Heel Spur Ostectomy (Open Method)
- ☐ Heel Spur Ostectomy (Rasping Method)
- ☐ Peroneal Tuberosity Recanalization
- ☐ Dwyer's Osteotomy

HALLUX VALGUS SURGERY

- ☐ Jones Operation
- ☐ McBride Operation
- ☐ Kaplan Operation
- ☐ Silvers Operation
- ☐ Lapidus Operation
- ☐ Reverdin Operation
- ☐ Akin Operation
- ☐ Keller Operation
- ☐ Mayo Operation

WEDGE OSTEOTOMIES

- ☐ Metatarsal, etc.

ARTHRODESING PROCEDURES

- ☐ Phalangeal
- ☐ M.P.J.
- ☐ Mid-Tarsal
- ☐ Sub-Talar

FRACTURES

- ☐ Phalanges
- ☐ Metatarsal
- ☐ Mid-Tarsal
- ☐ Calcaneus
- ☐ Talus

IMPLANTS

- ☐ Silastic
- ☐ Metal

- ☐ Privileges Granted
- ☐ To be reconsidered

Signed: ______________________________
Chief of Podiatry Service

Signed: ______________________________
Administrator

Date: ______________________________

To allow anyone to perform surgery because he is a friend or a favorite colleague would be catastrophic to the department.

This is not to imply that the surgeon in the reviewing stand is attempting to keep other podiatrists down. It is surely obvious that there are some podiatrists who do not have the talent or even the inclination to make the grade necessary to enjoy full privileges. Those who have the talent and the desire to advance their surgical privileges, however, should be helped and a method of evaluating their competence set up.

Surely, any ambitious, thinking podiatrist will desire to improve his status, learn the finer points of his profession, become more adept at them and open up a wider avenue of accomplishment for himself than he has heretofore enjoyed. For such dedicated practitioners, the doors must be fully opened and every opportunity for advancement in their specialized profession guaranteed them.

Special Equipment and Instruments for Podiatry Operations

Most hospital operating rooms are set up for orthopedic surgery and so have virtually all of the traditional equipment required, such as tourniquets, Kirschner wires, drills, osteotomes, plaster of Paris splints, etc. What are usually lacking are the special instruments normally used by the podiatric surgeon.

Since podiatric surgery usually includes bone and joint surgery in very small and important joints, good instrumentation is vital if the surgery is to be effective.

There is an old adage which says that instruments do not a surgeon make but it is just as true that

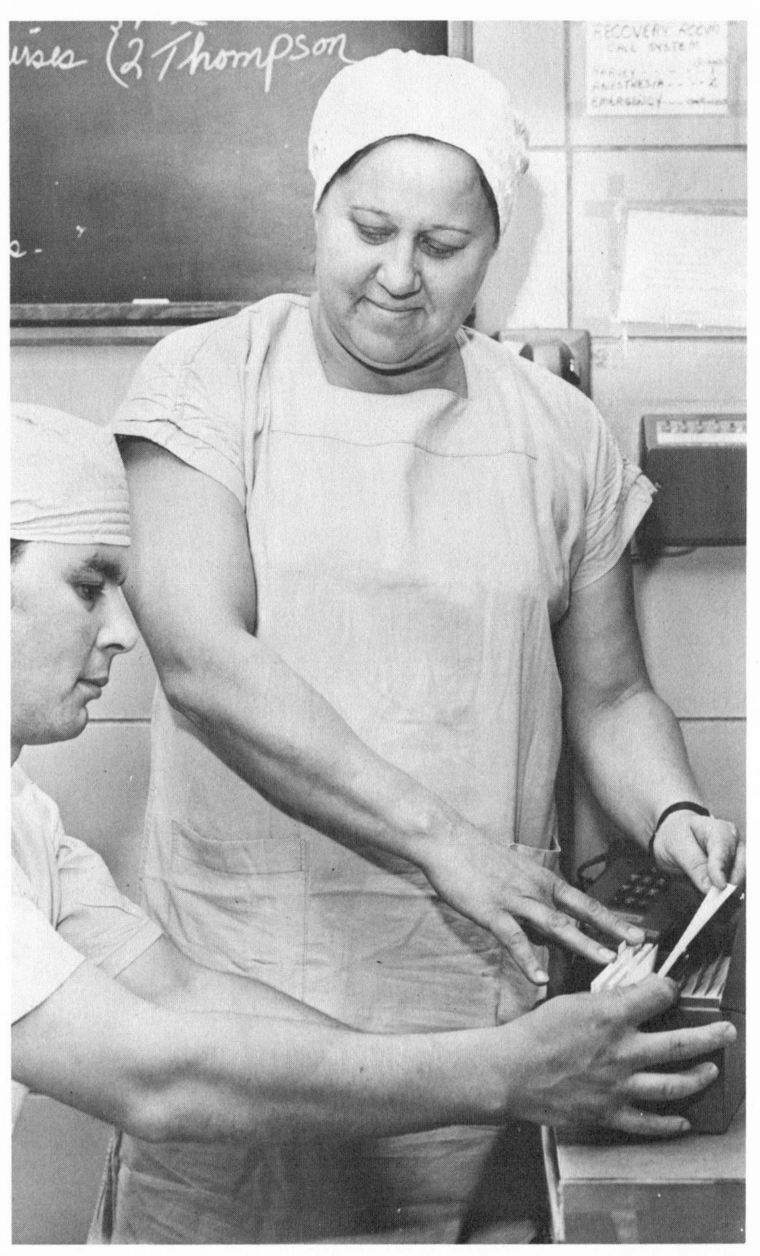

The chief of podiatric surgery reviews a control card with the OR supervisor. This is an important safeguard to insure adequate peer review, prior to surgery.

good instruments will make the most of his existing talents.

It is vital that you purchase the finest quality surgical instruments from a reputable house that will guarantee their product. Any supply house will gladly show you their line of instruments. Take your time and pick instruments which feel comfortable in your hands. This is particularly true of a needle holder or a bone mallet.

Following herewith, is a list of these articles you will require:

2 #3 knife handles
1 straight scissors
1 collar and crown scissors
2 curved mosquito hemostats
2 straight mosquito hemostats
4 Allis forceps
4 Babcock forceps
2 needle holders
2 baby towel clips
1 thin periosteal elevator
1 large rasp
1 small rasp
2 osteotomes (large and small)
1 mallet (large)
1 Curved tip bone forceps
2 thumb and finger forceps
1 Weitlander retractor
2 Seeburger retractors
2 15″ pieces of #3 orthopedic stockinette
2 2″ Kling bandages

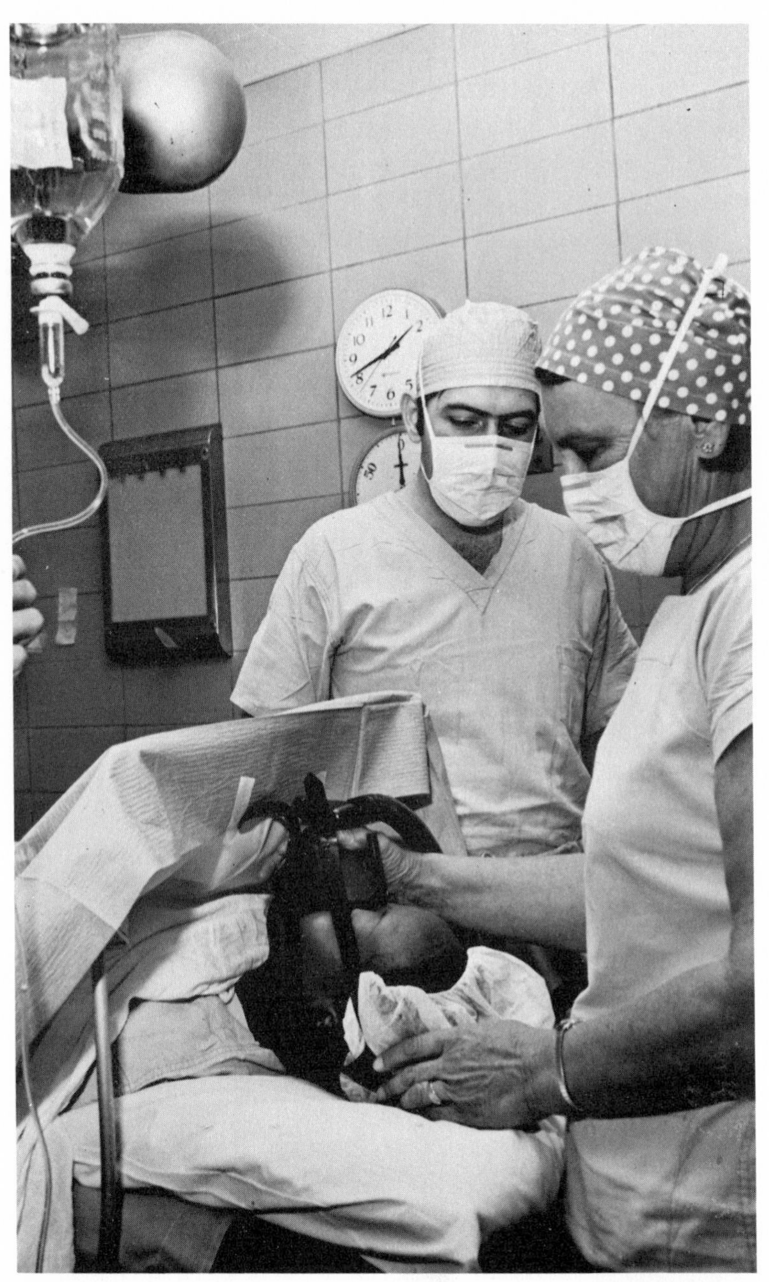

The patient is readied for anesthesia by the nurse anesthesist and the podiatric anesthesia residents.

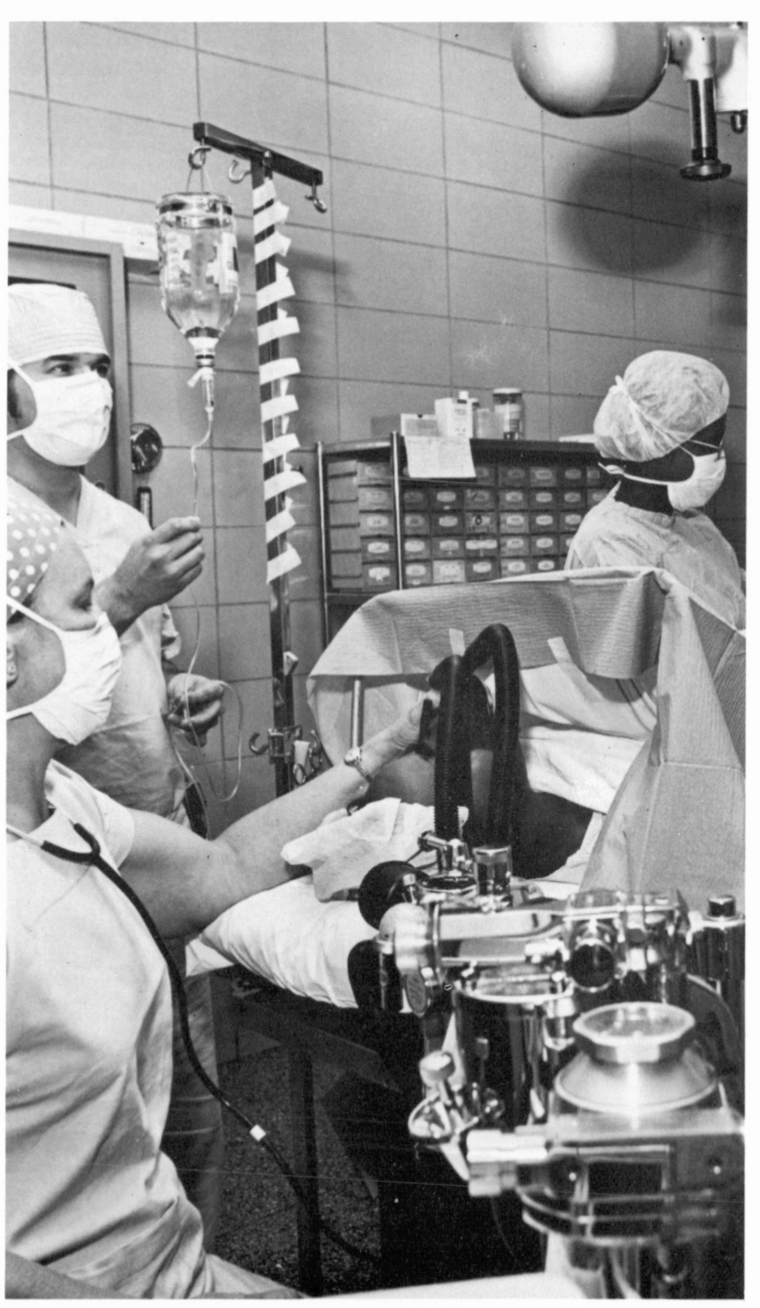

Once the patient is anesthesized, preparations for the operation begin.

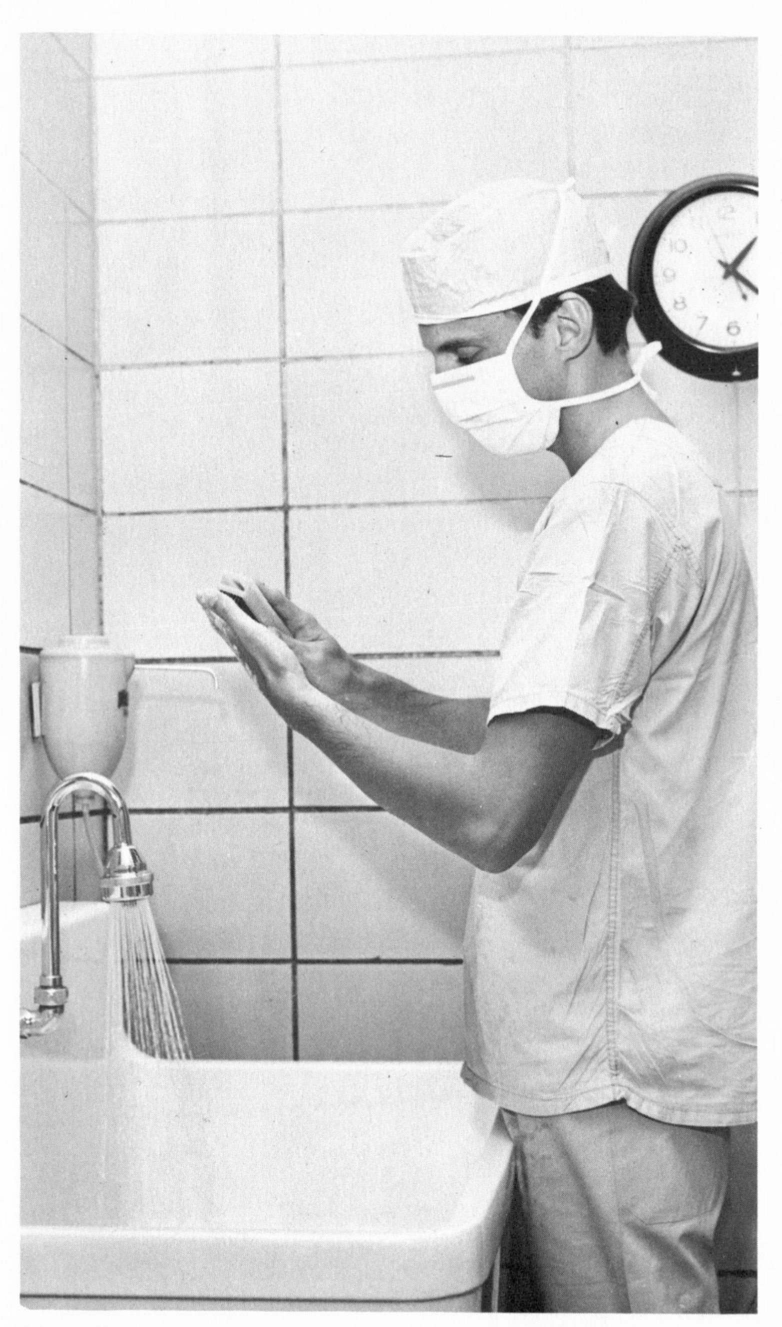

The podiatric surgeon scrubs in preparation for the surgery.

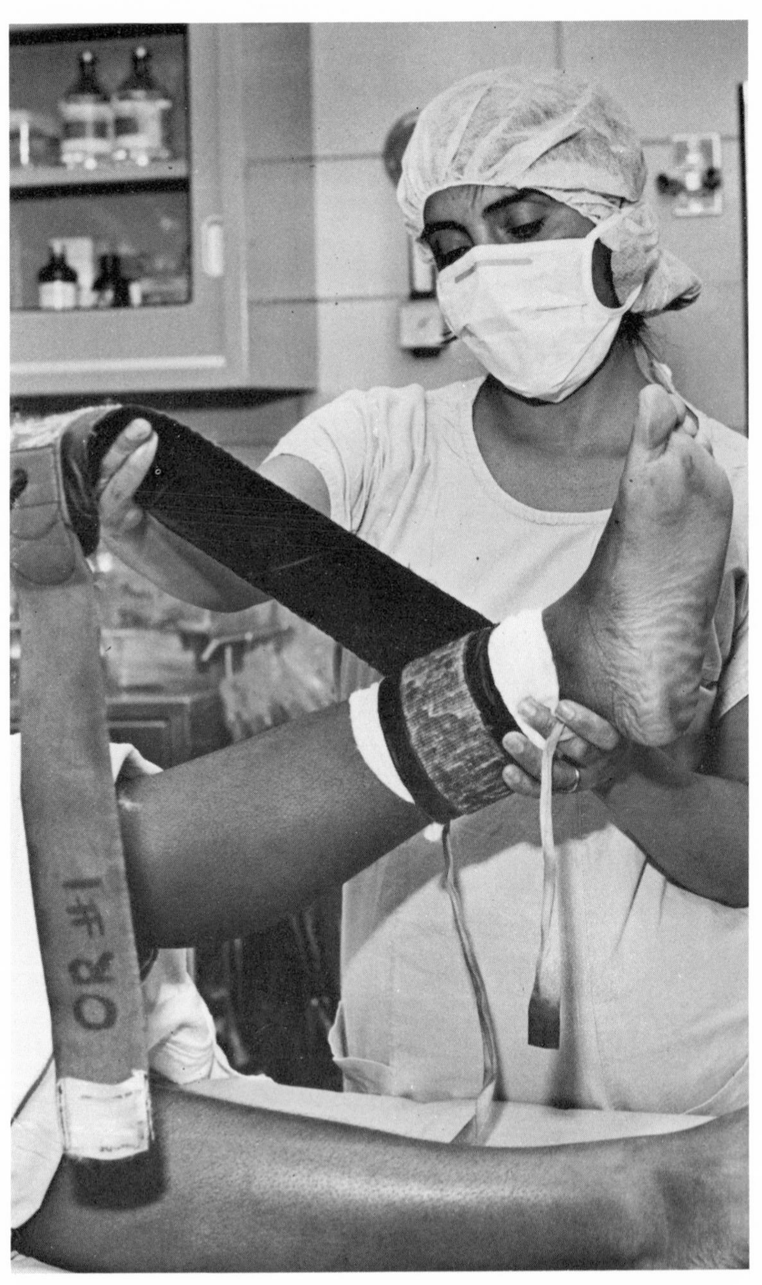

A pneumatic tourniquet is applied to the patient's leg to insure adequate hemostasis.

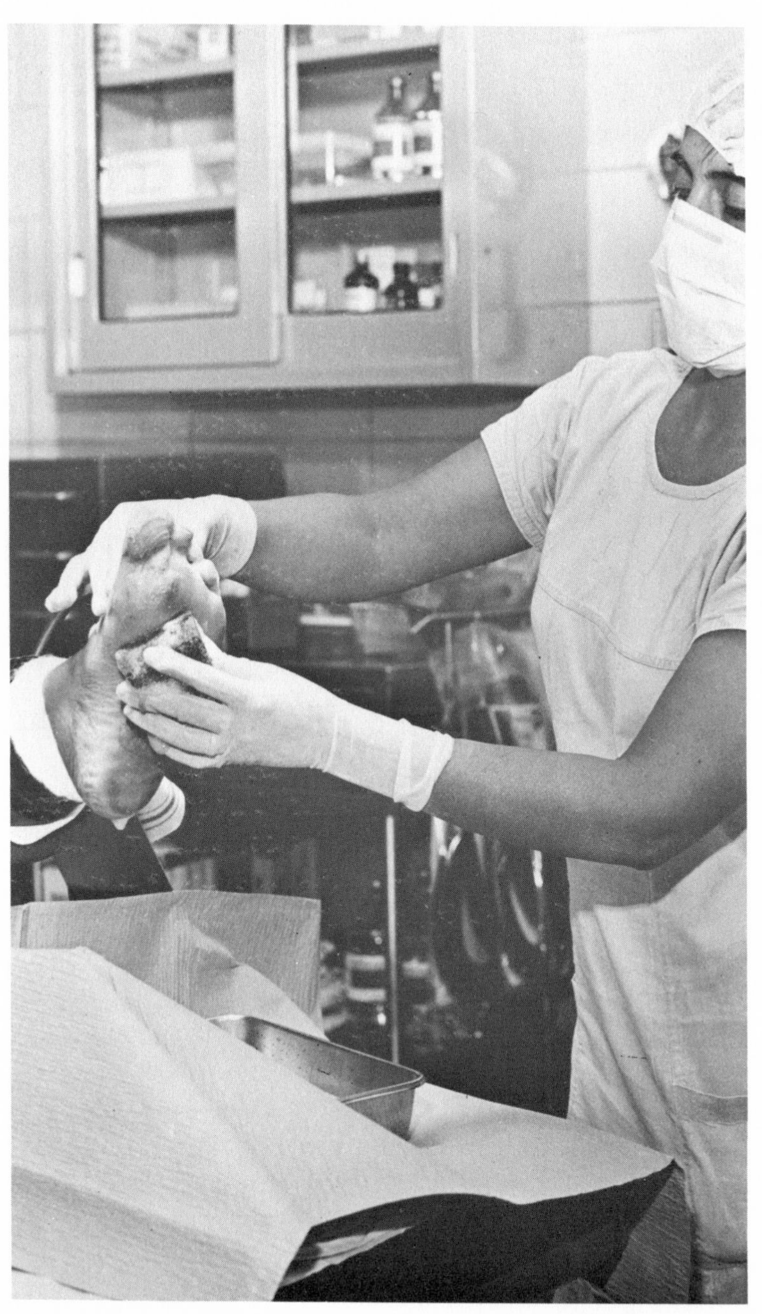

The circulating nurse scrubs the foot in preparation for the surgery.

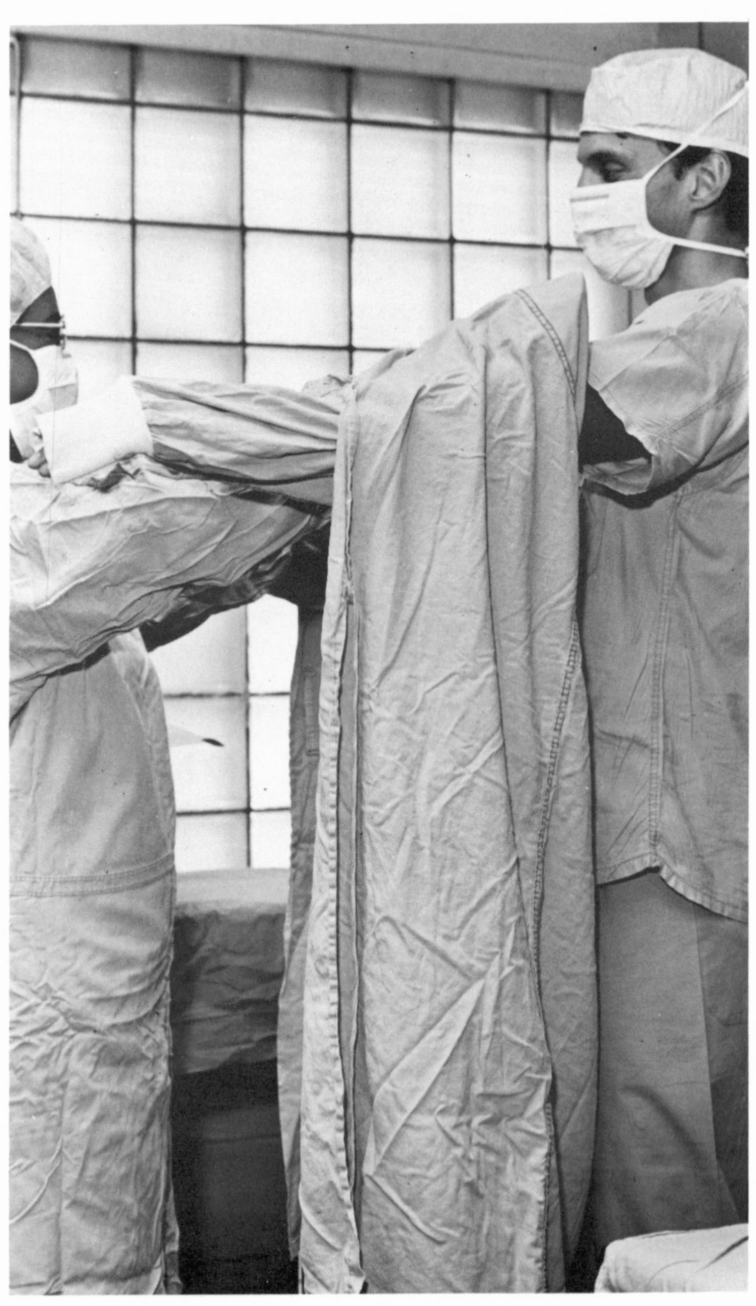

The podiatric surgeon is helped into his gown by the scrub nurse.

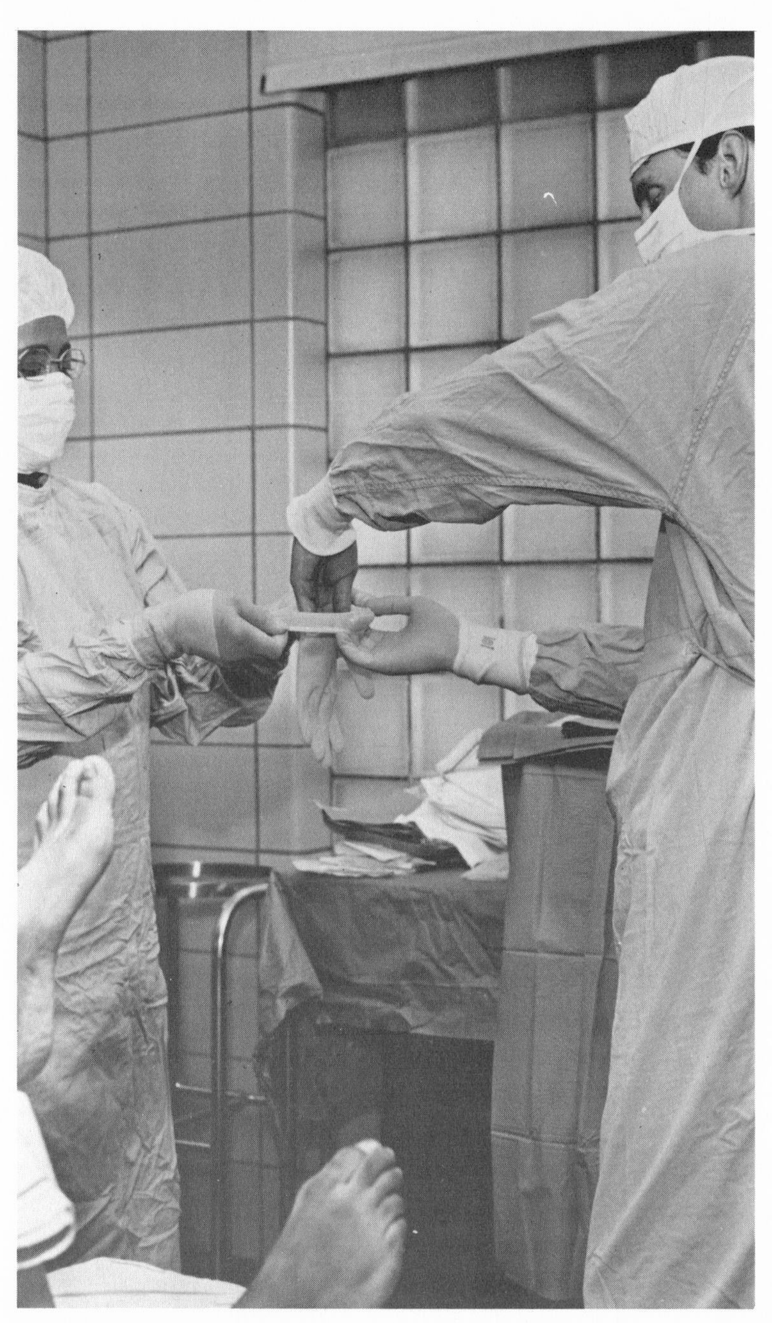

The surgeon is adequately gloved.

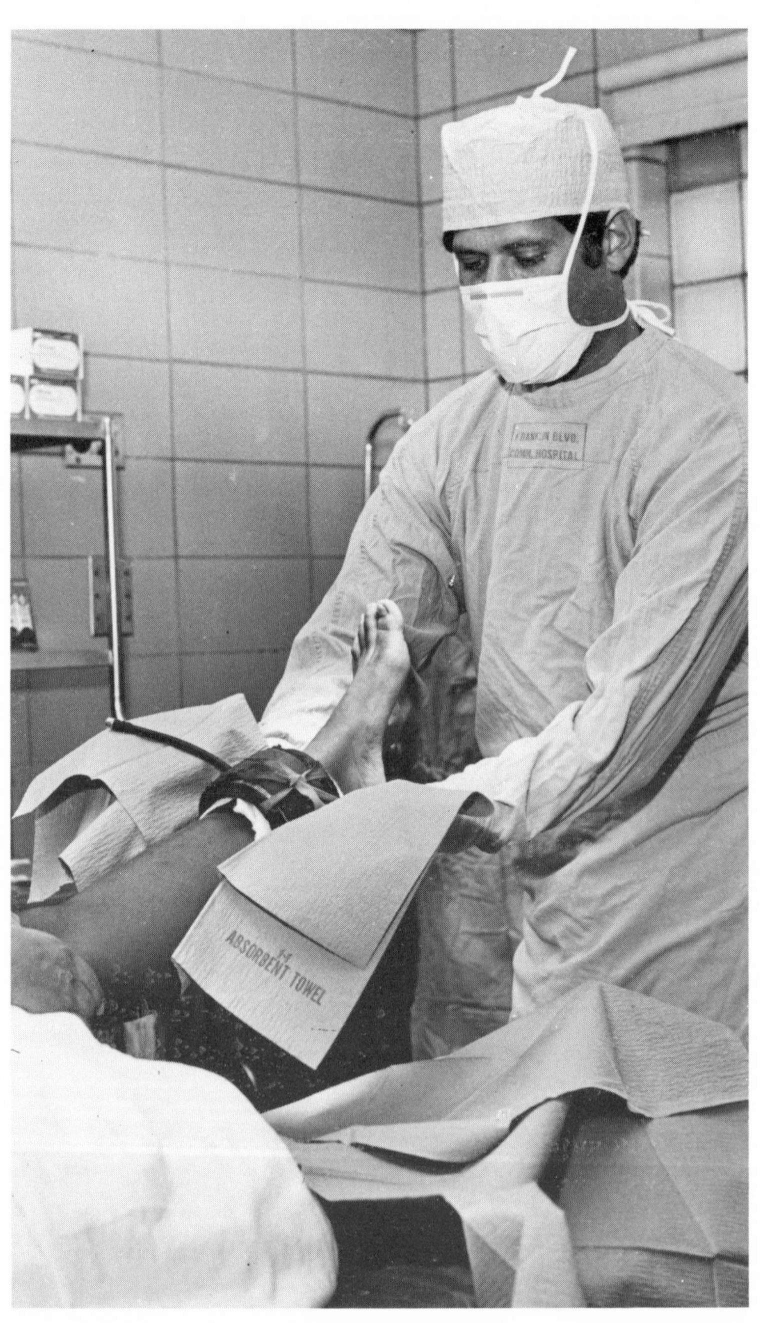

The assistant surgeon drapes the foot.

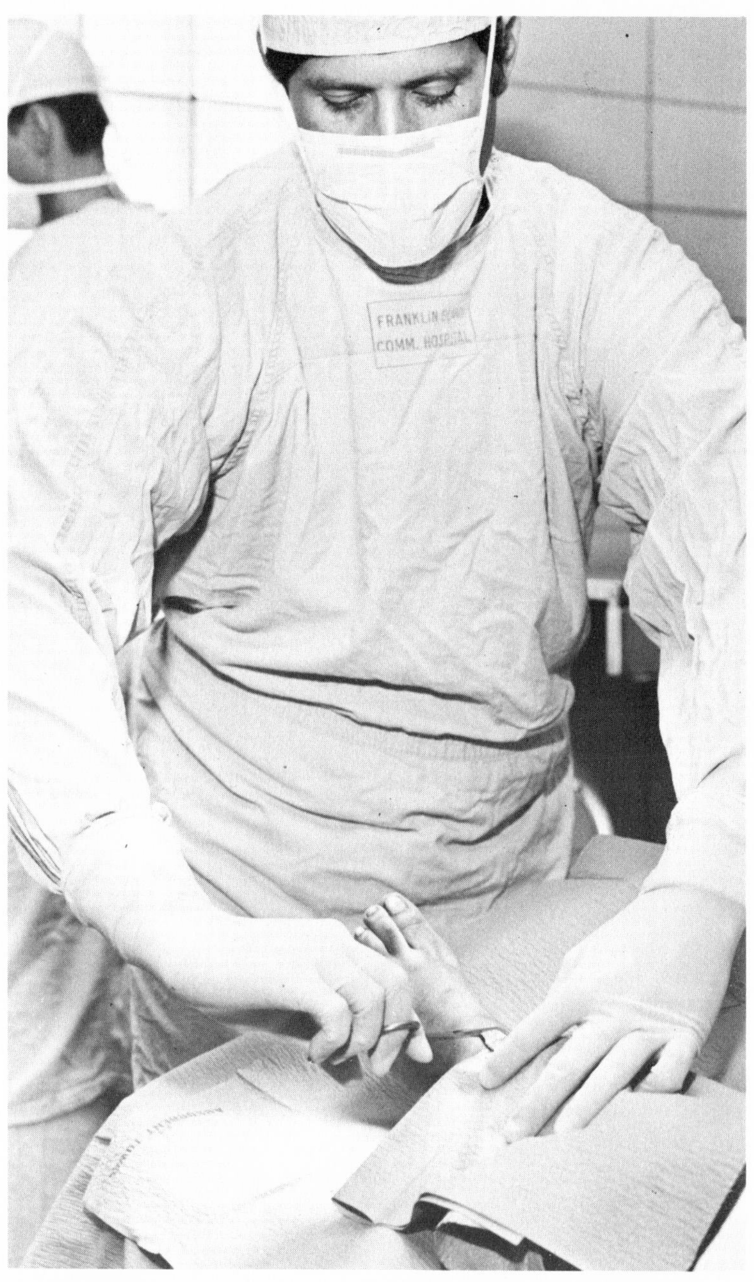

It is important to segregate the foot with sterile drapes to insure adequate sterility.

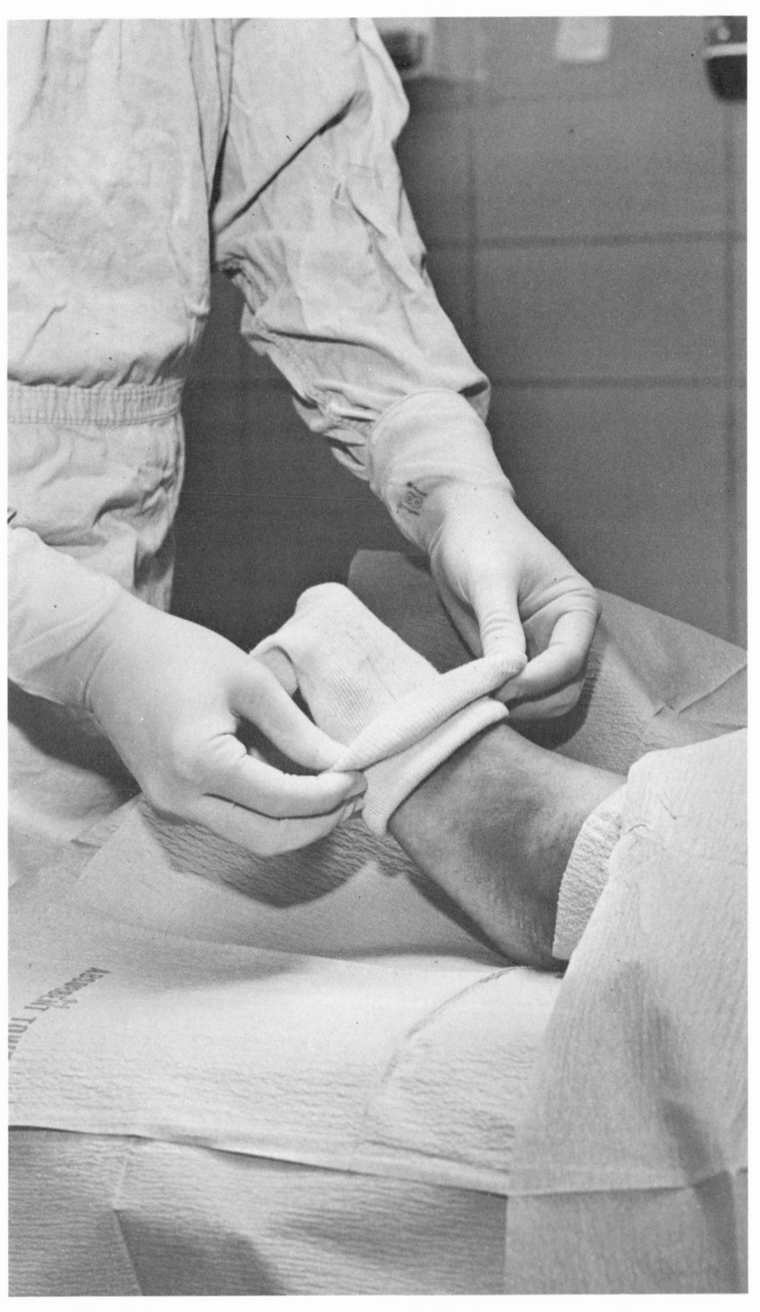

A stockinette is applied over the foot to insure an aseptic field.

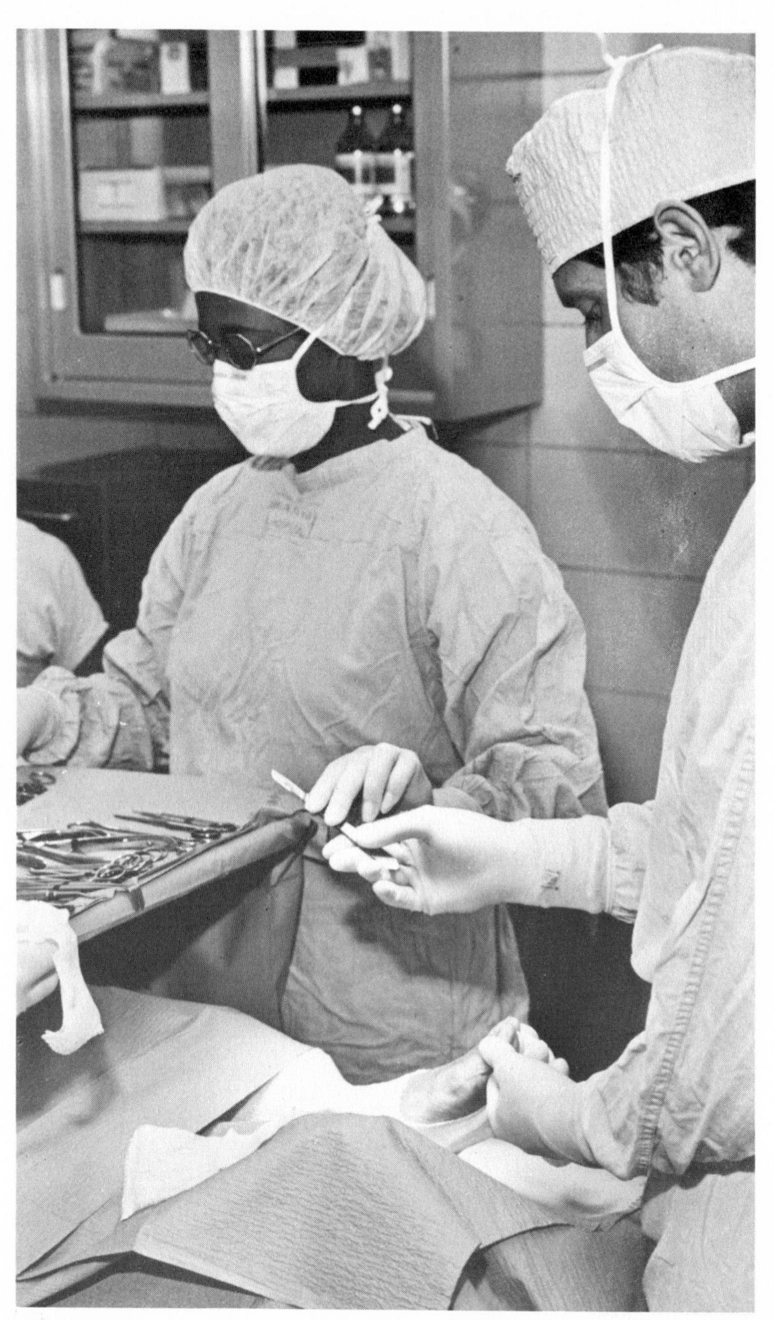

The surgeon is now ready to begin the operation.

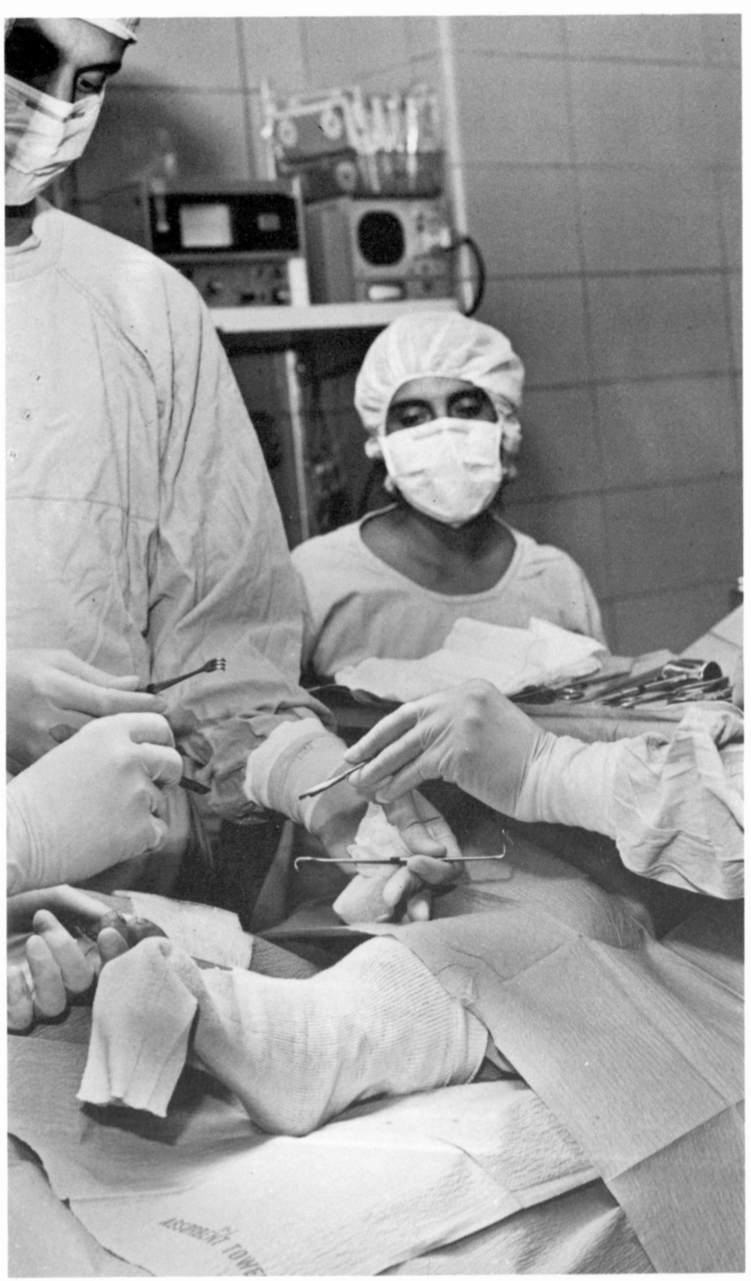

There is nothing quite as magnificent in the health picture as an OR team that works together as a single unit. . . .

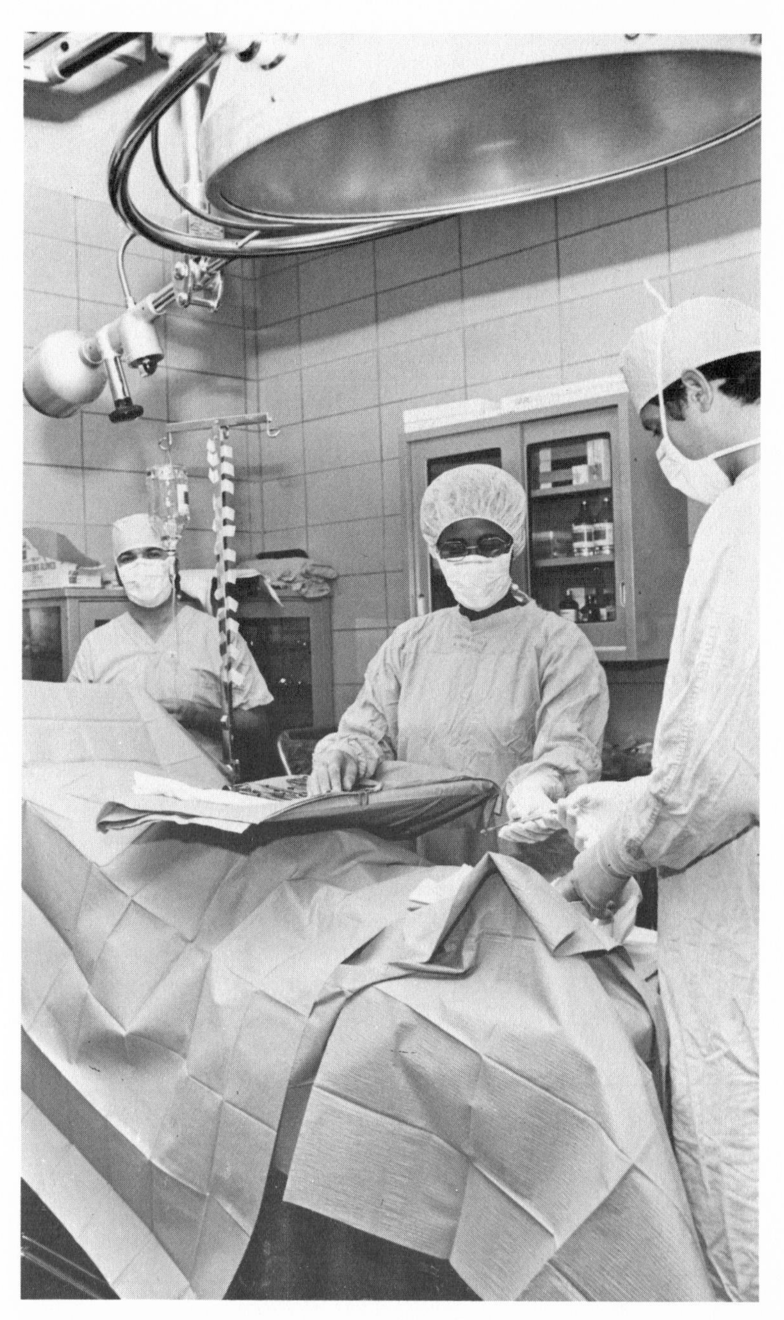

To insure the best possible overall care for the patient.

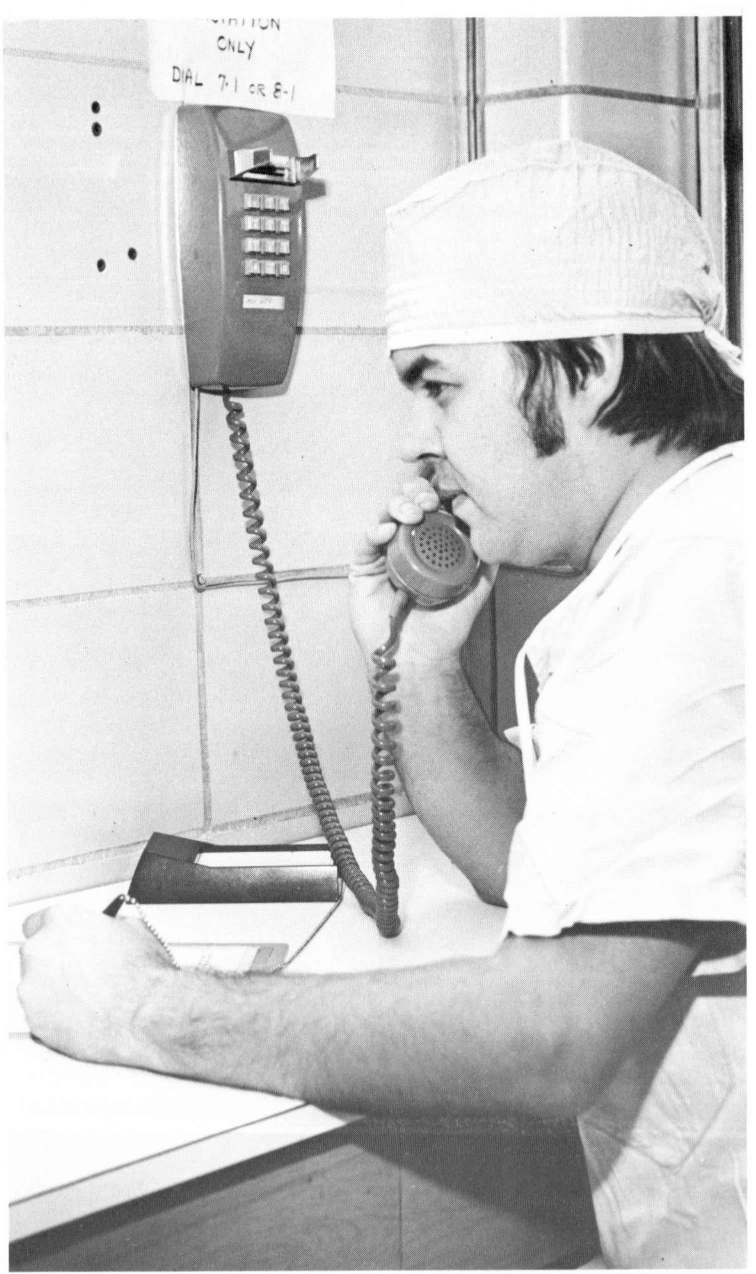

The podiatric surgeon dictates the operation report immediately after the surgery.

Hospital Protocol

The medical student is so trained that hospitals and hospital protocol are part of his educational environment. In podiatry, it has only been recently that the training of podiatrists emphasized hospital training and protocol. As a result, the average podiatrist may be totally familiar and competent in his own office practice but would be somewhat at a loss when functioning in a hospital atmosphere.

Hospital protocol is nothing more than good manners. Since hospitals are essentially public institutions, they have certain rules and regulations that must be followed by every member of the hospital medical staff, nurses, administration and all the way through to Housekeeping.

Let us take a sample, John Doe Community Hospital as an **ideal** institution where podiatric services are included. The following pages define the definition and by-laws under which it might operate and explains clinical privileges, podiatry services and protocol for the practitioner who would be working there:

THE JOHN DOE COMMUNITY HOSPITAL

Preamble

BECAUSE the John Doe Community Hospital is a non-profit organization organized under the laws of this State, and

BECAUSE its purpose is to serve as a general community hospital providing patient care, education and research; and

BECAUSE it is recognized that the medical staff is responsible for the quality of medical care in the hospital and must accept and discharge this responsibility, subject to the ultimate authority of the hospital governing body, and that the cooperative efforts of medical staff, the chief executive officer and governing body are necessary to fulfill the hospital's obligations to its patients;

THEREFORE, the physicians, dentists, and podiatrists practicing in this hospital hereby organize themselves into a medical staff in conformity with these bylaws.

DEFINITIONS

1. The term "medical staff" means duly licensed medical physicians and osteopathic physicians, and duly licensed dentists and podiatrists are priv-

ileged to attend patients in the hospital.

2. The term "governing body" means the governing board of the hospital.
3. The term "executive committee" means the executive committee of the medical staff unless specific reference is made to the executive committee of the governing body.
4. The term "chief executive officer" means the administrator appointed by the governing body to act in its behalf in the overall management of the hospital.
5. The term "practitioner" means an appropriately licensed medical physician, an osteopathic physician or an appropriately licensed dentist or podiatrist.
6. The term "service" means that group of practitioners who have clinical privileges in one of the general areas of medicine, surgery, dentistry or podiatry.
7. The term "chief of service" means the medical staff member duly appointed or named in accordance with these bylaws to serve as the head of a service.

ARTICLE I: MEMBER IN MEDICAL STAFF

Section 1. Nature of Medical Staff Membership

Membership on the Medical Staff of The John Doe Community Hospital is a privilege which shall be extended only to professionally competent practitioners who continuously meet the qualifications, standards and requirements set forth in these bylaws.

Section 2. Qualifications for Membership

a. Only physicians, dentists, and podiatrists licensed to practice in this State, who can document their background, experience, training and demonstrated competence, their adherence to the ethics of their profession, their good reputation, and their ability to work with others, with sufficient adequacy to assure the medical staff and the governing body that any patient treated by them in the hospital will be given a high quality of medical care, shall be qualified for membership on the medical staff. No physician, dentist or podiatrist shall be entitled to membership on the medical staff or to the exercise of particular clinical privileges in the hospital merely by virtue of the fact that he is duly licensed to practice medicine, dentistry or podiatry in this or in any other state, or that he is a member of some professional organization, or that he had in the past, or presently has, such privileges at another hospital.

b. Acceptance of membership on the medical staff shall constitute the staff member's certification that he has in the past, and his agreement that he will in the future, strictly abide by the Principles of Medical Ethics of the American Medical Association or by the Code of Ethics of the American Dental Association or by the Code of Ethics of the American Podiatry Association, whichever is applicable.

Section 3. Conditions and Duration of Appointment

a. Initial appointments and reappointments to the medical staff shall be made by the governing body. The governing body shall act on appointments, reappointments, or revocation of appointments only after there has been a recommendation from the medical staff as provided in these bylaws; provided that in the event of unwarranted delay on the part of the medical staff, the governing body may act without such recommendation on the basis of documented evidence of the applicant's or staff member's professional and ethical qualifications obtained from reliable sources other than the medical staff.

b. Initial appointments shall be for a period extending to the end of the current medical staff year of the hospital. For the purposes of these bylaws the medical staff year commences on the 1st day of January and ends on the 31st day of December of each year.

c. Appointments to the medical staff shall confer on the appointee only such clinical privileges as are specified in the notice of appointment, in accordance with these bylaws.

ARTICLE II: CATEGORIES OF THE MEDICAL STAFF

Section 1. The Medical Staff

The medical staff shall be divided into honorary, active, associate and courtesy staffs.

Section 2. The Honorary Medical Staff

The honorary medical staff shall consist of physicians, dentists and podiatrists who are not active in the hospital or who are honored by emeritus positions. These may be physicians, dentists, and podiatrists who have retired from active hospital practice or who are of outstanding reputation, not necessarily residing in the community. Honorary staff members shall not be eligible to admit patients, to vote, to hold office or to serve on standing medical staff committees.

Section 3. The Active Medical Staff

The active medical staff shall consist of physicians, dentists, and podiatrists who regularly admit patients to the hospital, who are located closely enough to the hospital to provide continuous care to their patients, and who assume all the functions and responsibilities of membership on the active medical staff, including where appropriate, emergency service care and consultation assignments. Members of the active medical staff shall be appointed to one or more services, shall be eligible to vote, to hold office and to serve on medical staff committees, and shall be required to attend medical staff meetings.

Section 4. The Associate Medical Staff

The associate medical staff shall consist of physicians, dentists, and podiatrists who are being considered for advancement to membership on the active staff. They shall be appointed to a specific service and shall be eligible to serve on committees of their services and to vote on matters before such committees. They shall be ineligible to hold office in the medical staff organization, however they shall be eligible to vote for officers of the medical staff at the annual election.

Section 5. The Courtesy Medical Staff

The courtesy medical staff shall consist of physicians, dentists, and podiatrists who are qualified for staff membership but who only occasionally admit patients to the hospital or who act only as consultants. They shall be appointed to a specific service but shall not be eligible to vote or hold office in the medical staff organization. They shall be eligible for appointment to the Professional Activities Committee and the Utilization Review Committee.

Section 6. All Initial Appointments are Provisional

All initial appointments to any category of the medical staff shall be provisional until the end of the medical staff year. Reappointments to provisional membership may not exceed one full medical staff year, at which time the failure to advance an appointee from provisional to regular staff status shall be deemed to termination of his staff appointment.

ARTICLE III: CLINICAL PRIVILEGES

Section 1. Clinical Privileges Restricted

a. Every practitioner practicing at this hospital by virtue of medical staff membership or otherwise shall, in connection with such practice, be entitled to exercise only those clinical privileges specifically granted to him by the governing body, except as provided in Sections 2 and 3 of this Article III.

b. Every initial application for staff appointment must contain a request for the specific clinical privileges desired by the applicant. The executive committee's evaluation of such requests shall be based upon the applicant's education, training, experience, demonstrated competence, references and other relevant information, including the appraisal of the applicable service(s). The applicant shall have the burden of establishing his qualifications and competency in the clinical privileges he requests.

c. Periodic redetermination of clinical privileges and the increase or curtailment of same shall be based upon the direct observation of care provided, review of the records of patients treated in this or other hospitals and review of the records of the medical staff which document the evaluation of the members' participation in the delivery of medical care.

d. Privileges granted to dentists shall be based on their training, experience and demonstrated competence and judgment. The scope and extent of surgical procedures that each dentist may perform shall be specifically delineated and granted in the same manner as all other surgical privileges. Surgical procedures performed by dentists shall be under the overall supervision of the chief of surgery. All dental patients shall receive the same basic medical appraisal as patients admitted to the other surgical services. A physician member of the medical staff shall be responsible for the care of any medical problem that may be present at the time of admission or that may arise during the hospitalization.

e. PODIATRY SERVICES

(1) Hospital Privileges. The governing body of the hospital, on recommendation of the medical staff, shall grant a qualified po-

diatrist privileges within his area of practice. The medical staff must evaluate the qualifications of each podiatrist who applies for hospital privileges after the recommendation of the podiatry committee.

The degree of privileges accorded each podiatrist must be determined by his professional education, training, experience, competence, and his demonstrated character and judgment. A podiatrist with hospital privileges may initiate the admission of a patient with the concurrence of a member of the medical staff, but no admission may be completed without such concurrence. The medical staff member concurring in a patient's admission assumes responsibility for the overall care of the patient including the medical history and physical examination. When podiatric surgery is indicated, the member of the medical staff may assume supervision of the podiatric surgery. The nature and degree of his participation is a matter for his determination in each case within the general policy adopted by the medical staff governing the relationship and dual responsibility between the physicians and the podiatrists. The podiatrist may write orders within the scope of his license as limited by the applicable statutes and the hospital regulations.

(2) Patients admitted to the hospital for podiatric care must be given the same careful medical appraisal as those admitted to other services. This makes the care of the podiatric patient the dual responsibility of the

podiatrist and the physician. Policies concerning the admission and discharge of a podiatric patient is determined by the medical staff and clearly stated in the bylaws. Every podiatric inpatient must have a physician with appropriate medical staff privileges who is available and will be responsible for the overall aspects of the patient's care throughout the hospital stay.

(3) An applicant for podiatric privileges shall have the same general type of qualifications as those outlined by the medical staff. A podiatrist is a graduate of a school of podiatry approved by the Council on Education of the American Podiatry Association and legally licensed to practice podiatry in this State.

(4) The podiatrist shall conform to standards established for the medical staff and shall be governed by the same ethical and moral codes and by the Principles of Ethics of the American Podiatry Association.

(5) The terms and procedures of an appointment shall be the same in general as those outlined for the medical staff.

(6) The podiatrist shall conform to the Rules and Regulations of the medical staff with the following additions:

(a) As in all surgical cases, an adequate medical history and physical examination by a member of the medical staff and podiatrist shall be required on each patient before surgery. Consultation with the medical staff shall be required when medical complications are present. A qualified member of the medical staff must be responsible for the care of any medical problems that may be present or arise during hospitalization.

(b) Complete records, both podiatric and medical, shall be required on each patient and shall be part of the hospital record.

(7) The podiatric staff shall select one member who shall act as the chief of podiatry. He shall represent the podiatric staff as a member of the executive committee, and shall report directly to the Chief of Staff of the medical staff on all matters relating to podiatric medicine.

* * * *

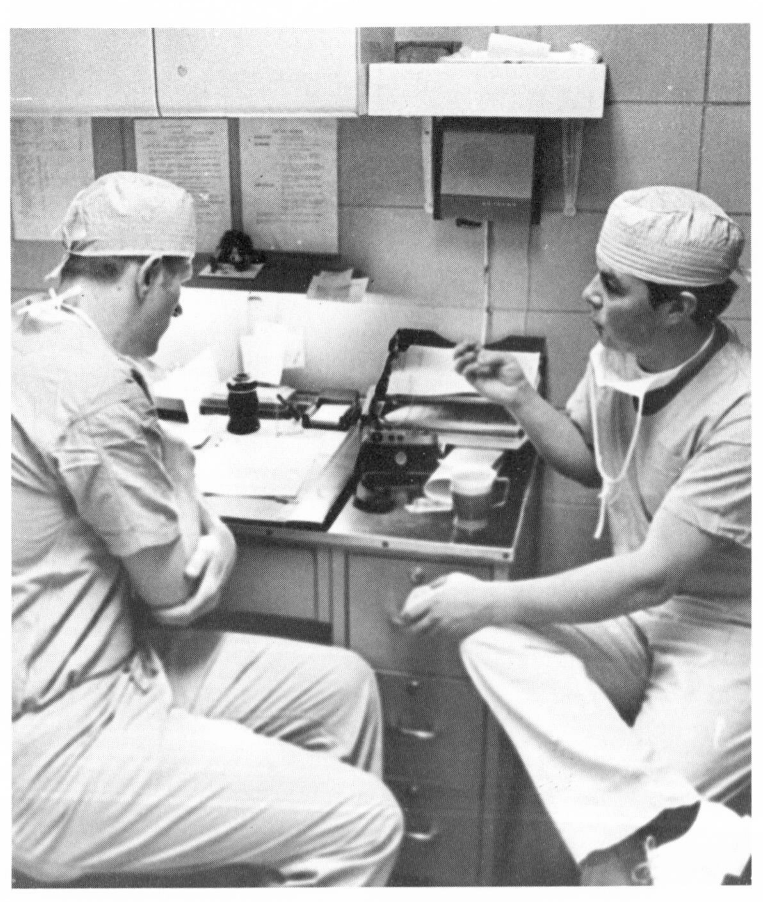

Two podiatric surgeons review a difficult case prior to operating. It is this intimate case discussion which makes hospital podiatry unique and effective.

Pre-operative Orders in the Hospital

Pre-operative orders seem to be routine and this may create false impressions. The orders are made to fit the patient. The patient is not made to fit the orders. Some of the orders may appear to be insignificant but they are all equally important in preparing the patient for surgery.

A list of fifteen pre-operative orders has been developed here. Of course, we do not use all of them for every patient and we add others depending on the patient and the type of anesthesia to be given.

1. Patient to operating room ______________ (time and date). When the time is not known, "Patient to operating room when called for" is written.
2. Oral hygiene at P.C. and hs. (The main reason for this order is to have the mouth clean and to protect the anesthesiologist against patient halitosis.)
3. Turgex bath at hs. (Any antibacterial soap may be used and the reason is self-explanatory.)
4. Turgex foot soaks at 4:00 PM and 8:00 PM and then at 5:30 AM. Place feet in sterile towel. (Patient soaks feet 20 minutes at three different times before going to surgery. This is one reason for low percentage of infection. The last foot soak is given one-half hour before the premedication is administered.)
5. NPO after midnight. (If the patient is under 14 years of age, night feeding at hs and the NPO after midnight is ordered.)

6. Fleets enema if no BM today. (If patient is 15 years of age or younger, a child fleets enema is ordered. For those patients over 50 years of age, a TWE (tap water enema) is ordered, because the Fleets enema is too irritating to the older patients' colons.)
7. General Diet (A specific diet such as diabetic, low-fat, or specific calorie diet will be given according to the physical needs of the patient.)
8. Patient to be ambulatory. (If this order is not written, the patient will be confined to his bed.)
9. X-rays: AP, lateral and oblique bilateral. (Additional x-rays may be ordered depending upon the patient's pathology.)
10. Inapsine 5 mg IM at 6:00 AM. (This sedative, anti-emetic agent is given two hours before surgery. Following trials of various other drugs, we found this drug to be more satisfactory for the patient's need before surgery.)
11. Meperedine 75 mg IM at 7:00 AM. (This narcotic is given one hour before surgery for analgesic purposes, and wll raise the patient's pain threshold 60 to 65%.)
12. Atropine 0.4 mg IM at 7:00 AM. (This drug is given one hour before surgery to inhibit the secretory glands in the oral and nasal passages, as well as in the tracheal-bronchial tree.)
13. Dalmane 30 mg cap at hs. (This is given to ensure the patient a good night's sleep, making the patient more cooperative and easy to work with the morning of surgery. We have tried other sedatives such as nembutal, placidyl, sodium seconal, etc., but have found Dalmane superior.)
14. BP both arms in PM and early AM. (This will enable us to get a better understanding of the patient's blood pressure. Often the patient is very

nervous at the time of examination and this may give us a false impression of his real blood pressure.)

15. ECG and PFT and place results on chart before patient goes to operating room. (Everyone over the age of 35 or anyone who shows cardiac pathology upon examination should have an electrocardiogram. Everyone over the age of 50 or who smokes 20 or more cigarettes a day or shows pulmonary pathology upon examination should have pulmonary function tests.)

The above orders do not include CBC, VDRL, urinalysis, FBS, SMA-12 and chest x-ray which are routine for all surgical candidates except for children in whom VDRL and chest x-ray may be excluded.

Summary

These pre-operative orders give us a sedated, cooperative patient the day of surgery. Again, we must emphasize that the orders are made for the patient and one should not get into the habit of following a fixed routine.

Post Operative Orders with General Anesthesia

The following are a list of post-operative orders that we use at Franklin Boulevard Community Hospital:

FIRST DAY:

1. Vital signs prn until stable then every 2 hrs x 4.
2. Patient to hyperventilate turn, cough every 2 hrs while awake.
3. Bedrest today.
4. Elevate feet on pillows and foot cradle for bed.

5. General diet and liquids as tolerated post-nausea.
6. Morphine SO_4 10 mg IM every 3-4 hrs prn for pain.
7. Inapsine 5 mg IM every 6 hrs prn for restlessness or nausea.
8. Placidyl 500 mg orally at hs (Patient over 50).
9. Nembutal 100 mg orally at hs (Patient under 50).

SECOND DAY:

1. D/C Morphine SO_4.
2. Demerol 50-100 mg every 3-4 hrs prn for pain or Darvon c ASA i tab 3-4 times a day for pain.
3. Bathroom privileges (BRP) with walker.
4. Medium sized surgical shoes.

THIRD DAY:

1. Continue Darvon c ASA.
2. Post-operative X-rays AP & Lat Oblique of feet.

Post Operative Orders When Perfusion Anesthesia Issued

FIRST DAY:

1. Bital signs q 15 min until stable then q 2 hrs x 4.
2. Bedrest today.
3. Elevate feet on pillows and foot cradle for bed.
4. General diet and liquids as tolerated post-nausea.
5. Morphine SO_4 10mg IM every 3-4 hrs prn for pain.
6. Inapsine 5mg IM q 6 hrs prn for restlessness or nausea.
7. Placidyl 500mg orally at hs (Patient over 50). Nembutal 100mg orally at hs (Patient under 50).

SECOND DAY:

1. D/C Morphine SO_4.
2. Demerol 50-100 mg every 3-4 hrs prn for pain or

Darvon—c ASA 1 every 3-4 hrs for pain.
3. Bathroom privileges (BRP) with walker.
4. Medium sized surgical shoes.

THIRD DAY:

1. Continue Darvon c ASA.
2. Post-operative X-rays AP & Lat Oblique of feet.

Post Operative Orders When The Spinal Anesthesia is Used

FIRST DAY:

1. Vital signs prn until stable then every 2 hrs x 4.
2. Patient to continue IV drip, 1000cc of Normal Saline for next 8 hrs.
3. Bedrest today.
4. Elevate feet on pillows and foot cradle for bed.
5. General Diet and liquids as tolerated post-nausea.
6. Morphine SO_4 10 mg IM every 3-4 hrs prn for pain.
7. Inapsine 5 mg IM every 6 hrs prn for restlessness and/or nausea.
8. Placidyl 500 mg orally at hs (Patient over 50). Nembutal 100 mg orally at hs (Patient under 50).

SECOND DAY:

1. D/C Morphine SO_4.
2. Demerol 50-100mg every 3-4 hrs prn for pain or Darvon c ASA 1 every 3-4 hrs for pain.
3. Bathroom privileges (BRP) with walker.
4. Medium sized surgical shoes.

THIRD DAY:

1. Continue Darvon c ASA.
2. Post-operative X-rays AP & Lat Oblique of feet.

The Hospital Administration and the Podiatrist

The Administrator of a hospital is a competent and versatile man or woman, chosen by the Board of Trustees to be their chief executive officer. His duties are many and varied but his principal role is to provide first-class medical care for the patients of the community which his hospital serves.

The Administrator's secondary but equally important role is to administrate the hospital in such a manner that it will remain financially solvent. If he spends more than he takes in, if he permits leakage of funds, if through ignorance of proper administration he is constantly in the "red" then, indeed, he is headed for big trouble.

It is obvious that the role of Administrator in a good-sized hospital is crucial and difficult, for he must please a wide variety of people. He must provide his surgeons with the latest, most sophisticated equipment for their work but at the same time, make equally sure than his Housekeeping Department has the mops, cleaning fluid and linens they require to maintain a clean and aseptic hospital.

The Administrator is responsible to his governing board for the running of the hospital. He must please not only the doctors and surgeons on his staff but the Women's Auxiliary as well, which as is well known, is made up principally of doctors' wives. He must seek funds for special improvements needed by the hospital and adequately prepare for full accreditation by the Joint Commission, without whose approval his hospital cannot endure.

He has to keep his experienced and competent help happy and content—his nurses, technicians, staff workers. And, in addition to all this, he has the problems of a changing society, changing neighborhood and other disturbing urban developments which can and often do affect him adversely. He knows that if the neighborhood becomes run down he will have trouble attracting the kind of help which a hospital needs to do its work properly.

The Admnistrator is on call 24 hours a day. A disaster or an emergency will often get him up at odd hours of the night. He strives through frequent disaster and fire drills to make his employees capable of handling emergencies but, for the important happenings, he must be there. His is the final, authoritative word and it is sought by each of several hundred people who work for him.

How, then, does the Administrator, plagued by so

many arduous tasks, so much continuous work and detail, look upon podiatry? What would inspire him to introduce such a brand-new element into his hospital picture, especially when it is bound to bring problems with it? He is a realist, he knows the temper of his people and he is aware of the discussions, arguments and antagonisms which will ensue among staff members before the new section grooves in and becomes an accepted part of the hospital picture.

If he is a man who is afraid of even temporary dissension, if he is a man who would avoid bickering and trouble at any cost, if an eternal calm is his highest objective, then perhaps there is no place for a viable podiatry section in his institution. Anyone knows that no newcomer can invade an established field of endeavor without disrupting some routines, ruffling some feathers. He knows this to be inevitable.

On the other hand, the Administrator is aware that introduction of a competent podiatry section within his hospital will enable him to provide more complete, overall care for his patients. He also knows that such a move can be very profitable financially for his hospital. As we have noted in a previous chapter, the podiatry patient is normally a very good patient. His stay is usually quite brief, he requires minimal nursing care both pre- and post-operatively, and he utilizes the facilities of the laboratory, x-ray department, anesthesiologist, recovery room, pharmacy and other departments of the hospital at an excellent profit to the institution.

Unfortunately, there is another side to the ledger which we just touched upon previously. There is no question that a new podiatry section often creates resistance from members of the medical staff, many of whom do not recognize or accept the podiatrist as a specialist in his field; from the surgeons who do not wish to be preempted in the Operating Room; from the nursing staff who, having never been exposed to podiatry patients and their needs, may offer resistance to that with which they are unfamiliar; to the radiologist who is not accustomed to reading foot x-rays and is of times unsure of precisely what he is looking for.

However, no part of this situation is unsurmountable. The physicians on staff, once they see and realize that the modern podiatrist is a man of excellent medical training and very competent in his specialty, usually get over their dislike and often become very interested, not only in sharing notes and discussing cases with the podiatrist, but in lecturing the podiatric residents and in helping the department grow.

In similar fashion, the surgeon who may be in charge of the peer review mechanism to gauge a podiatric surgeon's competency, will most often be won over once he sees that the podiatrist is first-rate in surgery, a man as painstakingly trained and competent to do his job as he is himself. Likewise, the nursing staff is bound to be won over by the podiatrist's dedication, devotion and care for the patient and will eventually make friends with him.

There can be no question in the thinking Administrator's mind that, without a podiatry section, he cannot provide complete, overall care for his patients. If he has delayed for one reason or another, he must soon face up to the fact that more and more patients are demanding competent podiatric care and it is only a matter of time when he will be forced to include such a section in his hospital.

Beyond all this, is the stark and incontestable fact that no Administrator can pass up such a useful and profitable innovation in his institution. If he does not ride roughshod over his medical staff but explains the facts of life to them, it will not be long before they come around to his way of thinking. Hospital Administrators throughout the country have found that, although it was a battle to get the new department set up, in virtually every case it has proven gratifying, an improvement in overall health care as well as financially worthwhile.

The podiatrist approaching a hospital Administrator for help in setting up a podiatric section, must understand that this executive's view of the working of the hospital is necessarily an overall one, and that podiatry is only a segment of that plan, one spoke in the wheel. He must follow the advice and suggestions of the Administrator, which cannot be too far from his own thoughts, since both are professionals seeking the same goal.

The podiatrist who comes into a hospital, establishes a section and makes his department profitable and worthwhile, and does this without stirring up too many waves, will make a friend of the Administrator, one which will stand him in good stead in all difficult future situations.

It is a good thought for a podiatrist making a request to try and see the ultimate decision from the Administrator's point of view. He must be sure in making the request that it is not too far out or impossible for the Administrator to grant. Peace is important to the executive handling a complex organization and it is wise not to add to such an executive's traumas.

The thoughtful podiatrist will run a tight ship and avoid giving any more trouble to the Administrator than is absolutely necessary. Especially if he is chief of service, it is his responsibility to manage the affairs of the department so that they encroach on no other and interfere with no other. The Administrator and he will get along famously if he adheres to his responsibilities and does not become a problem to that overworked executive.

We believe that every responsible podiatrist who gains admission to a hospital and becomes the head or an important integral worker in that section, owes a debt to his fellow-podiatrists. What is this debt? He should establish so favorable a relationship with the Administrator of his hospital, that this individual will recommend a similar section to all his fellow Administrators, who do not have such a department in their institutions. In doing this, he pays his debt to the profession which is giving him an excellent career and a profitable livelihood.

Hospital Administrators are people. They react well to consideration, to courtesies rendered, to friendships offered. The most they require of any department head in their hospital is that he conduct his department competently, fulfill his responsibilities, do his share to keep the hospital solvent. If he accomplishes these things, he gives no headaches to the Administrator and he becomes a good and dependable friend, a much sought-after commodity in the social and career marketplace.

Problems in Hospital Podiatry

As a virtual newcomer to the hospital scene, podiatry has its fair share of problems. These problems can be divided into four segments, (1) a mistaken interpretation of the Joint Commission's favorable stand on podiatry in hospitals, (2) problems arising in the Operating Suite, (3) a lack of awareness among the medical staff as to the new status, quality and achievements of modern podiatry, and (4) problems arising from members of the podiatry section.

(1) Those who have read the Joint Commission's dictum understand that individual hospitals have the option of creating a section of podiatry within their institutional format if they so desire. The ruling also permits the individual hospital great latitude in the implementation of rules regarding the podiatrist's activities within the hospital.

The ideal situation would be one in which the podiatrist could co-exist with all the other departments of medicine on an equal footing. As far as rules are concerned, the practice of podiatry within the hospital is limited by the laws of the state regulating the practice of podiatry in that state and the individual competency of the practitioner.

The Joint Commission expects and, indeed, insists that the podiatric patient receive the same over-all care as any other patient in the hospital. However, in a number of cases, the podiatric patient has been required to pay an exhorbitant fee for the physical examination performed by the co-admitting physician. This has not made him feel good toward either the podiatrist or the hospital.

Another common misinterpretation of the Joint Commission's ruling results in the podiatrist not being allowed to practice surgery to the full extent of the law, even though he may be fully qualified. It is essential that hospitals adopt a peer review mechanism and then give the qualified podiatrist a free hand to practice his specialty.

The hospital that knowingly or unknowingly imposes unnecessary restrictions on the qualified members of a podiatry section harm not only themselves but the patients whom they are supposed to serve. It cannot be too greatly stressed that in every instance where hospital podiatry sections have been permitted to grow and expand, both hospital and patients have benefited immensely.

Perhaps the best advice that can be given any hospital Administrator is to choose his podiatric staff wisely and with discrimination, then permit them to move ahead without restrictions to build the section into a respectable and successful department of the hospital.

(2) There is no other area in a hospital where more problems will arise for the podiatrist than in surgery. The basic problem here is, of course, that the podiatric surgeons lack Board Certification. Because of this fact and because the hospital has no other way of qualifying a man, it is absolutely vital that they have a capable podiatric surgeon watch, assess and qualify these practitioners. We would like to suggest a few guidelines for them to use in selecting a chief of the podiatric section:

(a) Proven experience in surgery. This can be ascertained by the type of patients the man has, his years in practice and personal observation of the manner in which he handles varied kinds of cases. Ideally, the man should have served a podiatric surgical residency.

(b) The individual's standing in the profession is important. Is he the kind of man who has accepted the challenges of his profession, does he serve on various podiatric committees or organizations?

(c) Is he a man who has written articles or published papers on the developments in his field and has he lectured extensively before other podiatrists or groups on podiatric problems?

(d) Does he have any teaching appointments? While this is desirable, we do not wish to be unfair. There are only five colleges teaching podiatry in the United States and his opportunities in this direction would be extremely limited.

3. One of the most difficult challenges to the hospital podiatrist is the lack of knowledge on the part of the medical staff as to the recent advances in podiatry and its present respectable standing among the professions. Too often, the physician's knowledge of the field is very antiquated and behind the times and his attitude, therefore, biased. There are some physicians who are unaware that there are podiatrists who can and do operate on their patients. The young podiatric surgeon, just completing his residency, who applies for admission to a hospital and then clashes head-on with one of these types, has a problem indeed—he really does!

The nursing staff can also be a source of problems if they are prejudiced and have no knowledge of a podiatrist's requirements. The veteran nurse who has never been exposed to podiatry will often look upon the podiatrist as someone akin to a technician and not particularly worthy of her respect. It is very important that the practicing podiatrist win over these nurses and this can be done better by deeds than by words.

Remember that the veteran nurse's image of a physician is one of a dedicated individual whose principal and abiding interest is the welfare of his patients. When she is made to realize that the podiatrist has the same identical interest, it will be easier for her to accept him.

(4) Thus far, we have discussed the trials and tribulations of the podiatric section emanating from the hospital in general. But how does the chief of the podiatric service handle the problem podiatrist, the man who is always late for surgery, never completes his records on time, dresses shabbily or indifferently,

in short, is the "enfant terrible" of the department?

We have heard some stories of podiatry sections which have failed to gain hold and even been closed due to the actions of such an individual. Unfortunately there is no easy, sure-fire way to handle him. It is essentially up to the chief of Podiatry. After consultation with the other members of his staff, and assembling of all the grievances, he must approach this individual and lay the law down to him. He must stress that when this podiatrist does the wrong or objectionable thing, the whole section is besmirched and suffers from his wrongdoing. The medical staff not only looks upon him as a bad egg, they look down at the whole department.

The podiatric chief must inform the erring podiatrist that his every action is having a bad effect on hospital personnel; that, in effect, he is doing an ill turn to all his fellow practitioners. He must be told that his careless conduct must stop or he will be removed from the staff forthwith.

It happens on occasion that a misfit of this type is a close friend of the Chief of Podiatry, which makes it extremely difficult for him to censor the culprit. If the podiatrist finds that he is not up to handling this assignment, he should appoint a small committee of the staff to do it.

One last word on peer mechanism. Look for it, anticipate it, ask for it. Not only does it win for the podiatrist permission to perform to the full extent of his capabilities but it also sees to it that those in practice who are not up to the highest standards of the profession, reach that plateau before engaging in this practice.

The Co-Admitting Physician

The Joint Commission on Accreditation of Hospitals requires that all entering podiatric patients be co-admitted by a staff physician. The staff physician's responsibility is to take care of the medical problems of the patient while the podiatrist takes care of his own specialized area.

There is no situation which has brought more dissension to the hospital podiatrist than a misunderstanding of the functions of the co-admitting physician, yet the purpose of having the co-admitting physician is really for the protection of both the podiatrist and the hospital.

Actually, the hospital wishes to assure the podiatric patient that he will receive as good medical care as any other patient who is admitted and that is the reason why this examination is done by a qualified staff physician. Another duty of the staff physician is to medically evaluate the patient's need and fitness for surgery. He makes certain that the patient is healthy enough to withstand the podiatric procedures.

When a co-admitting physician functions well, the quality of the care is unsurpassed. The diabetic patient who requires surgery can be assured that, not only will it be performed properly, but his medical condition will also be taken care of. This applies as well to hypertensive patients, rheumatoid, cardiac, etc.

The Joint Commission's ruling never intended the role of the co-admitting physician to be one of policing the podiatrist or limiting him. Unfortunately, in rare instances, the co-admitting physician has increased his authority and become tyrannical to the extent that the podiatric section becomes subservient to him. Sometimes his fee was out of line with the services provided and he occasionally came to consider podiatric patients as an excellent source of "beefing" up his account. Situations such as this, however, are very infrequent, and when they happen, they should be contested by the practicing podiatrist.

Now, let us clear up a point once and for all. The podiatrist has the legal responsibility for his patient and he does not lose this responsibility by taking his patient into the hospital. In fact, the malpractice insurance carrier for the American Podiatry Association provides an option which is called a "hold harmless option", which provides that, in the event a podiatrist is sued for surgery that he has performed, the podiatry association insurance will cover the co-admitting physician, since he is **not** responsible for the surgery. It is important that every podiatrist in hospital service carry this insurance because, in the eyes of the law, the podiatrist has the responsibility for that patient.

Unfortunately most insurance companies will not cover for the co-admitting physician fee. All patients should be told of the fee prior to being admitted so that they are totally aware of it.

In a sense, the podiatric patient is being castigated by the addition of a physical examination fee. The average medical patient is usually given the physical examination history by the hospital residents at no extra cost. In the case of the podiatric patient, the co-admitting physician has this duty to perform and he **must** be compensated for it. Perhaps in the future, the insurance companies and the hospital will find it possible to take care of this extra fee now paid by the podiatric patient.

Unlimited Licensed Practitioners

The term "unlimited license" has been used indiscriminately by the medical profession. In describing the scope of their practitioners, much discussion has been held over the fact that the podiatrist has a limited license only while the state gives the physician the legal right to do anything from extracting teeth to neurosurgery. But medicine has set up guidelines and criteria to limit the scope of it specialists, in order to assure the public that whoever is performing a specialty, is duly qualified. This means that the general practitioner is definitely limited to the scope of procedures that he can perform. So, really, in a practical sense, the podiatrist is no more limited in his specialty than the average physician.

GEORGIA STATE MEDICAL EXAMINATION GIVEN TO PODIATRISTS

Gordon E. Duggar, D.P.M. and E. Dalton McGlamry, D.P.M., reported in the August, 1973 issue of the Journal of The American Podiatry Association, that they gave the Georgia State medical examination to a group of podiatry residents and found that they acquitted themselves exceedingly well in this strictly medical quiz. The two Georgia podiatrists stated, "it should be no surprise that the podiatrists who took this examination did so well because, for quite some time, colleges of podiatric medicine have required the same basic medical education as is given in schools of medicine".

With postgraduate training for podiatrists increasingly rapidly, with study programs extending two and three years beyond the D.P.M. degree, a new horizon is emerging for the podiatrist. Indeed, the modern podiatrist has become a well-trained medical specialist, fully capable of functioning in the same manner as other specialists. Perhaps this mode of training podiatrists may suggest a better way to train other practitioners of diverse specialties within the medical arena.

There is a strong and growing feeling in the podiatry field that experienced podiatrists should be permitted to perform a history and physical on their own patients since this technique is taught in their colleges. Then they could eliminate calling in a consultant unless a medical problem should arise.

However, the weather vane turns, the up-to-the-minute podiatrist is happy to be a member of his hospital medical team, respectful of the knowledge, training and experience of his medical peers and glad to work with them in providing a more complete health service for the public they all serve.

Surgery and the Podiatrist

How does a podiatrist relate to the surgery department of a hospital where he serves? As is known, the podiatric surgeon comes under the rules of the department of surgery and he operates under the same strict regulations as any other surgeon.

In a previous chapter, we discussed the importance of properly qualifying the podiatric surgeon. We know that the privileges granted a podiatrist in the department of podiatric surgery are only those which he is held qualified to perform. We have also stressed the importance of frequent peer reviews of these qualifications to make certain that only fully qualified men perform surgery in the hospital. This ruling is no different for any other surgeon.

In every hospital setting, the functions of the podiatrist in surgery are actually more closely related to the orthopedic surgeon than to any other member of the medical team.

In his office, the podiatrist conducting a routine examination, will often uncover gait and other specific foot problems that are intimately related to the knee, the hip, the spine, and which require primary surgical care by the orthopedic surgeon.

For example, the parents of a young boy recently observed that their child was limping and took him to their podiatrist to see what could be done about it. A series of simple tests revealed that there was no foot problem per se, but that the child was actually limping because of a Legg-Perthes problem in his hip. The podiatrist then directed the parents to seek the services of a good orthopedic surgeon, competent in correcting such ailments.

Numerous patients come to podiatrists with foot problems which are directly related to neurosurgery, such as skeletal problems of the upper extremity. This trouble is reflected in the feet by revelation of improper balance and excessive fatigue factors. While it is an involvement related to the feet, it is also definitely a situation which logically requires surgical treatment by the orthopedic surgeon.

The pain often found by the podiatrist on, let us say, the medial aspect of the leg and ankle, may possibly be related to sciatic problems or lesions of the spinal cord, and this, too, falls entirely into the realm of the orthopedist.

In a hospital where a podiatrist is affiliated, the volume of foot surgery is increased from 100 to 500 percent. This takes nothing away from the orthopedic surgeons, indeed, the more cases the podiatrist handles, the more cases there are likely to be which call for referral to the orthopedic surgeon.

It is also a truism that when patients come to a hospital for podiatric care and later, become otherwise ill, they are very likely to come back to that hospital for treatment of their malady, especially if they liked the manner in which they were treated the first time. Anyway you look at it, treating podiatric patients in the hospital always proves a plus factor in increasing hospital business and medical referrals.

The Vascular Surgeon and The Podiatrist

Peripheral vascular disease is often manifested first in the lower extremities. The patient suffering with such a malady will come to the podiatrist's office, complaining of vague symptoms—numbness, coldness, general malaise. On examination, the competent podiatrist will find that some of the symptoms might be caused by vascular occlusions, ischemia, impending gangrene or any one of a host of other peripheral vascular problems, falling specifically into the realm of the vascular surgeon.

Often, being immediately referred to a competent vascular surgeon, has resulted in the saving of a patient's limb or even his life. One of the first suggested steps, after setting up a podiatric section in a hospital, is to have the vascular surgeon lecture the group on vascular diseases and how to recognize them. No other member of the surgical team will appreciate a podiatrist more than the vascular surgeon to whom such cases have been conscientiously referred.

In our hospital, the vascular surgeon has been an intimate segment of our teaching program. He lectures students and residents regularly and often has the residents scrub with him so that they can observe his techniques and learn from him. He has become one of the most verbal proponents of the profession of podiatry and has a real appreciation of the many cases discovered and referred to him by the podiatric staff. When an early diagnosis is made possible through the podiatrist's alertness, both doctor and patient have a better chance to treat the affliction successfully.

The General Surgeon and the Podiatrist

Surgery is surgery, no matter whether it is performed on the foot or the abdomen. The basics of the specialty are as essential to the surgeon as a pen to a writer.

There is no one more aware of the primary principles of surgery than the general surgeon. He can be of immense help to the podiatrist in giving him ideas on difficult surgical techniques, instrumentation or post-operative complications. His advice on difficult or perplexing procedures can be beyond price.

A story comes to mind of one of our staff podiatrists who, after groping around unsuccessfully for a foreign object, a needle in the foot, felt completely defeated and depressed—he could find nothing. Our senior general surgeon walked over and dryly welcomed him to the club, since he like many other surgeons, at one time or another, hopelessly looked for foreign objects in a patient and also failed to find them.

The surgeon then proceeded to induct the podiatrist in the basic premise that nothing is simple in surgery and the worst thing one can do is to underestimate the importance of any case. The podiatrist and the surgeon found an empathy in talking together and the end result was that the surgeon lectured the podiatrists and residents in the hospital and proved a deep well of knowledge.

The Pathologist and the Podiatrist

The field of clinical medicine has advanced more rapidly than perhaps any other field today. Tests which are now common were completely unheard of a few short years ago. Take the SMA 12/60. This marvelous machine performs 12 biochemical analyses simultaneously on each serum sample (720 determinations) per hour. Results are recorded automatically on precalibrated chart paper. These biochemical profiles give the physician immediate visual evidence of the performance of several organs. The biochemical profiling makes possible early diagnosis, more rapid initiation of appropriate therapy and the detection of unsuspected abnormalities before clinical symptoms develop.

The podiatrist should become familiar with the routine operation of the hospital laboratory where he works and know about the superlative aids to diagnosis and treatment which are available to him. He should meet and make friends with the chief pathologist, who will always be ready to share his knowledge and perception with the podiatrist, to the practitioner's great advantage.

It is also very important to talk with the pathologist about podiatric surgery. For example, one common procedure performed by the podiatrist is the resection of a neuroma. The podiatrist should explain the procedure to the pathologist so that he will know precisely what he is looking for when he examines his specimen.

Very often, in the case of some rasping techniques (osteotripsy), which is performed by podiatrists to reduce troublesome exostosis in the patient, a specimen of toothpaste-like residue is sent down to the lab for examination. The pathologist might really be baffled unless he was told how it was obtained and what information was required regarding it.

The Radiologist and the Podiatrist

The introduction of a new podiatry section in a hospital will be added work for the radiologist, who is often not used to examining x-rays of the feet. In the practice of podiatry it has become essential for diagnostic purposes, to obtain weight-bearing x-rays. If the radiology department is not advised of this, the x-rays will not be prepared properly. Also in many surgical procedures performed by podiatrists, such as ostectomies and osteotomies, it is difficult to see the actual work performed in post-operative x-rays, unless the radiologist knows what he is looking for.

In cases where bone disease or foreign objects are involved, the radiologist can offer the podiatrist a world of welcome information on how to proceed under varied circumstances. There is no question, the radiologist and the podiatrist can learn much from each other—and they should. Both will benefit from their admirable partnership.

The Anesthesia Department and Podiatry

Perhaps there is no department more important to the podiatric surgeon than the Department of Anesthesia. For many years, the podiatrist had to perform his surgery in his own office and could rely only on local anesthesia. With the advent of hospital podiatry, the practicing podiatrist has had made available to him a wide range of anesthesia techniques which he could freely utilize to make surgery easier for his patient as well as for himself.

It is well known that many patients refuse surgery in the office, even for minor procedures, because they are afraid of the pain. Now that this factor has been eased, the patient can be well pre-medicated and fully anesthetized, so that he need endure little discomfort. In a hospital, the patient with individual problems like diabetes, hypertension, cardiac malfunctions can be admitted well in advance of his surgery and be properly evaluated and treated prior to it.

In order for the podiatrist to relate well to the Anesthesia Department, he should make it a point to seek out the chief anesthesiologist and talk with him or her relative to any particular problems which might arise in foot surgery.

The anesthesiologist will be pleased to discover that most of the podiatrist's patients can be treated with just a light, simple anesthesia. As most podiatry procedures are of short duration, the anesthesia time will usually not be extended beyond the norm. In addition, the vast majority of podiatric patients are healthy patients with few if any disturbing medical complications.

Podiatric surgery lends itself to a great range of anesthetic agents. For example, all the standard gasses can readily be used. Even the newer forms of anesthetic agents, such as ketamine, can also be utilized for short procedures. Local anesthesia is useful when the general type cannot be employed on the patient. Local infiltration and nerve blocks which every podiatrist can perform himself, may be used at such times. In our hospital, our local blocks are potentiated with pre-medications; nitrous oxide and sometimes intravenous sedatives.

Perfusion Anesthesia

At Franklin Boulevard Community Hospital, we have successfully used perfusion anesthesia on hundreds of patients with consistently good results and few complications.

Essentially, perfusion anesthesia is nothing more than intravenous regional anesthesia. A double compartment cuff is placed on the patient's mid-leg, a

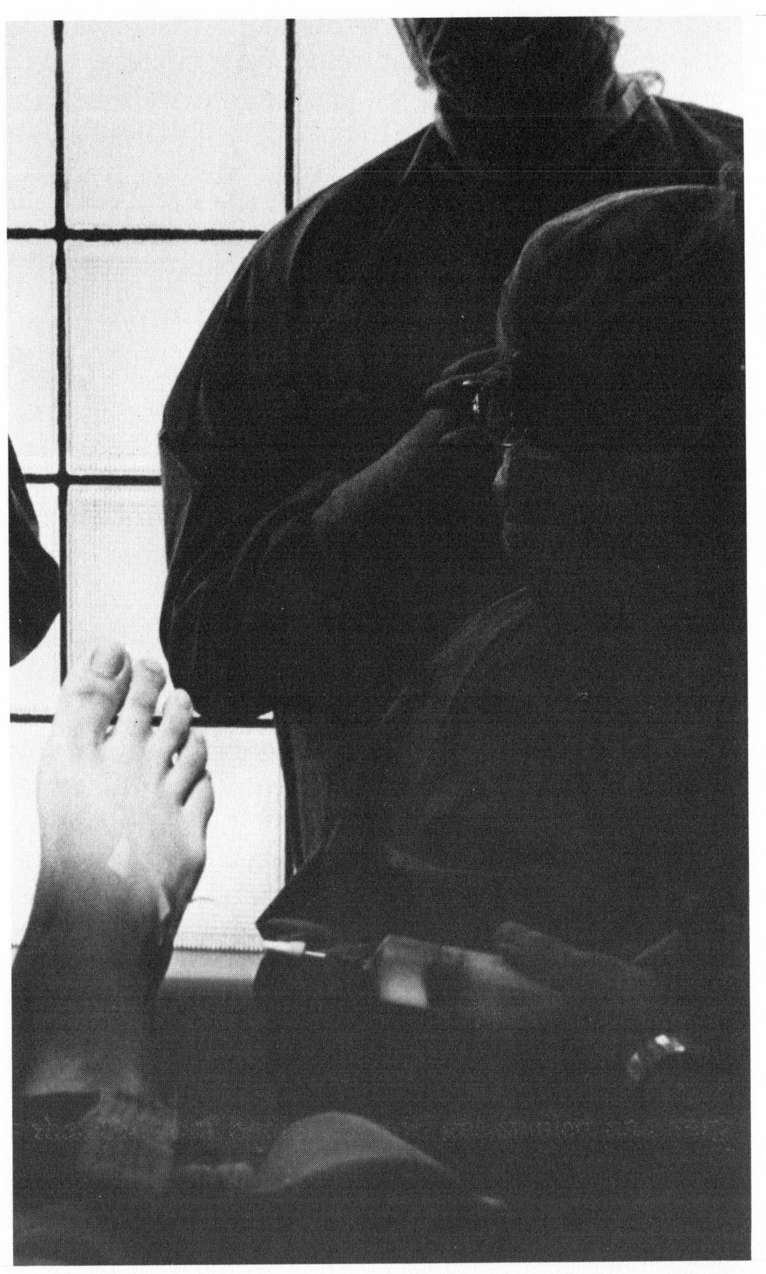

The perfusion anesthesia technique is demonstrated by the podiatric anesthesia resident.

PRN catheter is introduced into any available superficial vein. The leg is then drained for 5 minutes, then the upper compartment cuff is inflated to 300 mm/Hg pressure. Using 1% Lidocaine HCL, 2 mg's per pound of body weight is drawn on a 50 c.c. syringe (usually about 15-20 cc). Saline solution is then used to fill up the 50 c.c. syringe. This is then injected slowly into the veins. Blanching will occur and the anesthesia will be effective almost immediately.

If the patient complains of pain around the upper cuff area, then after 10 minutes, the lower cuff will be inflated with 300 mm/Hg and the upper cuff deflated. Since the area underneath the lower cuff has been anesthetized, the patient should experience no discomfort. The patient is then simply prepped in the usual manner and surgery can begin.

While perfusion anesthesia is old to medicine, its application to podiatry is new and credit for the development of its use in podiatry must go to Fern Sanner, M.D., Chief Anesthesiologist at Franklin Boulevard Community Hospital and Professor of Anesthesiology at the Illinois College of Podiatric Medicine. Dr. Sanner has also been responsible for preparing the anesthesia Questionnaire, for children and adults.

Filling out the Questionnaire properly is extremely important for the smooth running of a podiatric surgery department. There are many medications that a patient could be taking that will make it difficult to use normal types of anesthesia. As an example, the patient who has been on a long-term cortico-steroid therapy, must be prepared well before being submitted to the stress of anesthesia, since his adrenal glands will be unable to cope with the added stress, without supportive therapy.

CHILDREN

QUESTIONNAIRE FOR PROSPECTIVE CANDIDATES FOR GENERAL ANESTHESIA

NAME____

AGE____

SEX____

WEIGHT____________________HEIGHT____________________

PHYSICIAN'S NAME________________________________

PHYSICIAN'S ADDRESS______________________________

PHYSICIAN'S PHONE_______________________________

When was this child last seen by a physician?

Why

Date and nature of most recent illness.

Is this child taking any medication at the present time?

Past History	Date
Measles	
Mumps	
Chickenpox	
Other contagious disease, if any	
Croup	
Convulsions	
Rheumatic fever	
Diabetes	
Kidney Trouble	

Immunization History	Date
Vaccination for Small Pox	
Measles	
Polio	
Tetanus	
Diphtheria	
Whooping Cough	

Has this child ever been given cortisone? If so, when?

ADULT

QUESTIONNAIRE FOR PROSPECTIVE CANDIDATES FOR GENERAL ANESTHESIA

NAME____

AGE____

SEX____

WEIGHT__________________HEIGHT__________________

PHYSICIAN'S NAME______________________________

PHYSICIAN'S ADDRESS___________________________

PHYSICIAN'S PHONE_____________________________

1. When was your last illness?
2. What was wrong with you?
3. When was the last time you saw your family physician?
   Why?
4. Are you taking any medicine at the present time?
   If so, for what condition are you taking it?
   Give name of Medicine if known.
5. Have you ever had, or do you now have
   High blood pressure
   Arthritis
   Diabetes
   Bleeding tendency
6. Have you ever taken medicine for these conditions?
   When?

7. Are you allergic to any medicine? If so, what?

8. Do you require frequent rest periods when engaged in normal activity?

9. Do you become unduly fatigued after walking up a flight of stairs or wolking faster than usual?

10. Do you frequently experience shortness of breath?

11. Do you now experience or have you ever experienced any chest pain?

12. Do your ankles swell?

13. Do you have a cough?

14. Do you smoke? If so, how much?

15. do you drink? If so, estimate weekly usage.

16. Have you ever had an asthmatic attack?

17. Have you ever received an anesthetic? When?

18. Are you usually nervous? or have you ever had a nervous condition? When? Where?

Date: ____________________________
(Patient's Signature)

It is important in the case of patients with a questionable medical history, that the podiatrist get in touch with the patient's physician and ask his opinion as to whether the patient can withstand the surgery. In our experience in calling physicians regarding their patients, we have found them to be extremely courteous and helpful.

Besides the good public relations which results from the teamwork of podiatrist and physician, the benefit to the patient is of inestimable value. Actually, without this spirit of teamwork, the patient is the one who will suffer. The conscientious podiatrist will be more respected by his medical peers if he shows concern for the patient and a willingness to work as part of the medical team. Perhaps one should emphasize the point, that while we stress the importance of autonomy for the Department of Podiatry in a hospital, it is equally important that the podiatrist work within the framework of the medical picture. There can be no dichotomy.

The value of the above to the podiatrist is inestimable. Another outstanding way for him to build a successful podiatry section in a hospital is to make a real friend of the hospital anesthesiologist. He can lighten the podiatrist's load considerably and help insure the success of his surgical undertakings.

In our hospital, the residents rotate for six months in the Anesthesia Department. Here they learn everything from the intubation of the patient to the handling of medical emergencies. A program such as this helps make the podiatrist aware of the importance of proper training and patient care and the medical staff will look with more confidence on the podiatrist who has been properly trained.

As one of the physicians recently put it so well: "It is not that the podiatrist getting anesthesia training is a frustrated anesthesiologist, but rather that he is consistently being made aware of the importance of the over-all care of the patient and of his own significant role in the health picture".

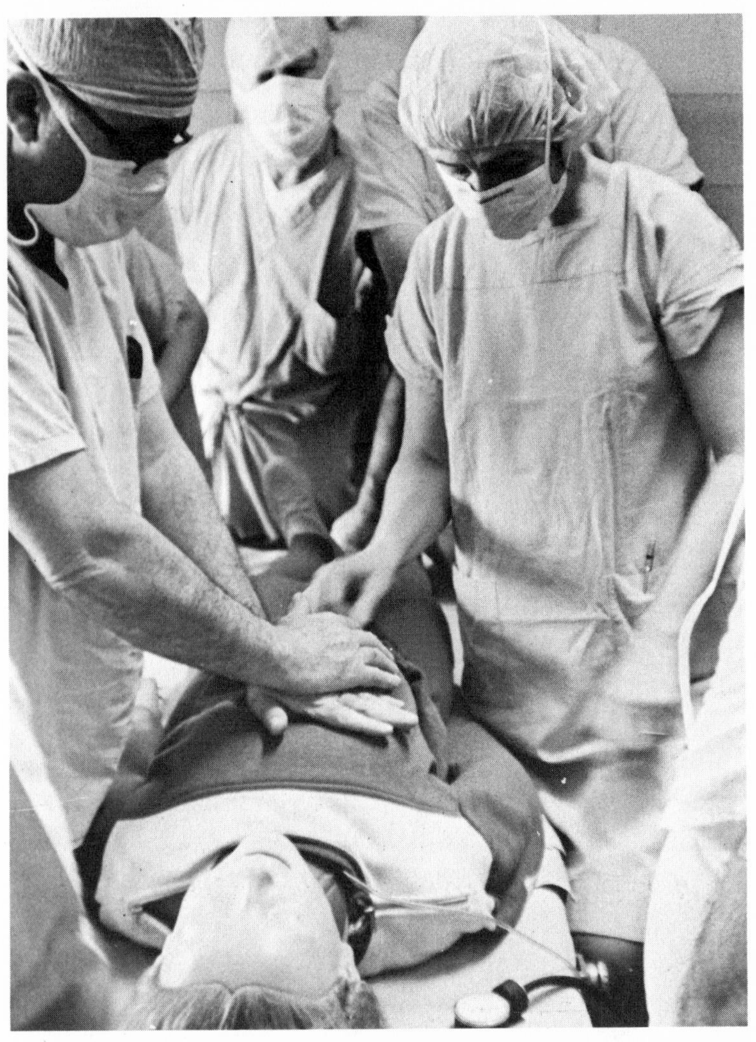

Podiatrists in postgraduate seminar review external cardiac massage under supervision of the anesthesiologist.

The Nursing Aspect of the Podiatric Patient

The average nurse, learning that a section of podiatry is soon to be opened in her hospital, might be concerned as to what is expected of her, especially if she has never had any experience with podiatry patients. She will be pleasantly surprised to learn that the average patient usually requires a minimum of medical or nursing care.

The podiatry patient is normally admitted to the hospital one day before surgery. That day, all of the standard lab tests are performed in addition to special x-rays of the feet. The patient is usually on a regular diet and is able to ambulate without assistance. The evening prior to surgery, the feet are scrubbed and draped and the patient is made N.P.O. after midnight. Usually, a sedative is provided for apprehensive patients.

The morning of surgery, the appropriate pre-operative medication is given as ordered by the Anesthesia Department. After surgery, the patient is usually placed in bedrest, with his feet elevated on pillows and a foot cradle attached to the bed. The only medication he might require is for pain, which will vary from patient to patient, and occasionally, medication for nausea.

On the day after surgery, the podiatry patient is usually allowed bathroom privileges with some assistance or the use of a walker. Also surgical shoes are ordered for him. In most instances, by the second day, post-op, the patient is comfortable, ambulating fairly well and ready to enjoy the cuisine and special services that every modern hospital provides.

Of course, it is entirely possible that complications might arise in a particular case which may require more intensive nursing care than usual, but this is the exception rather than the rule. The wise podiatrist will make friends with the nursing staff and talk over with the Nursing Director the various things his patient will require. As a rule, most hospitals have a supply of walkers and foot cradles although they might have to order an additional amount to meet their needs, once a podiatry section is established. Surgical shoes are also usually available in the hospital or they can easily be ordered from any medical supply house. The podiatrist should express his preference, since there are many available shapes and styles.

The dressings that are required by practicing podiatrists are also normally available on the nursing floor. These are 2-inch Kling bandages, 4x4 gauze pads, 3-inch Stockinettes, non-allergic tapes, usually a cortico-steroid spray and antibiotic ointments. If these are not available on the floor, they should be ordered promptly and in sufficient quantities so as to avoid frequent trips by the nursing staff to Central Supply.

The podiatrist should also talk over with the Nursing Director the rules and regulations regarding the plaster of paris casts, applications and removals. In many hospitals it is the policy that casts may be applied in the operating room only. If such is the case, the podiatrist should follow the ruling. Of course, if all he needs to do is to loosen the cast, this can certainly be done easily at the bedside by himself or any other member of the medical team.

The care provided by the nurses is of tremendous importance and the podiatrist will do well to work with the nursing staff and make friends of them. An excellent idea is to have a series of talks or lectures just for the nurses on the various aspects of podiatry, so that they may become more familiar with the field and its specialized techniques.

The Operating Room Nurse

The OR nurse is in a class by herself. She is the only person who can ease the burden of the podiatric surgeon's work through her valuable assistance, understanding, stamina and willingness to work hard under often difficult conditions.

What are the duties and responsibilities of an OR nurse? From the moment the patient comes into the

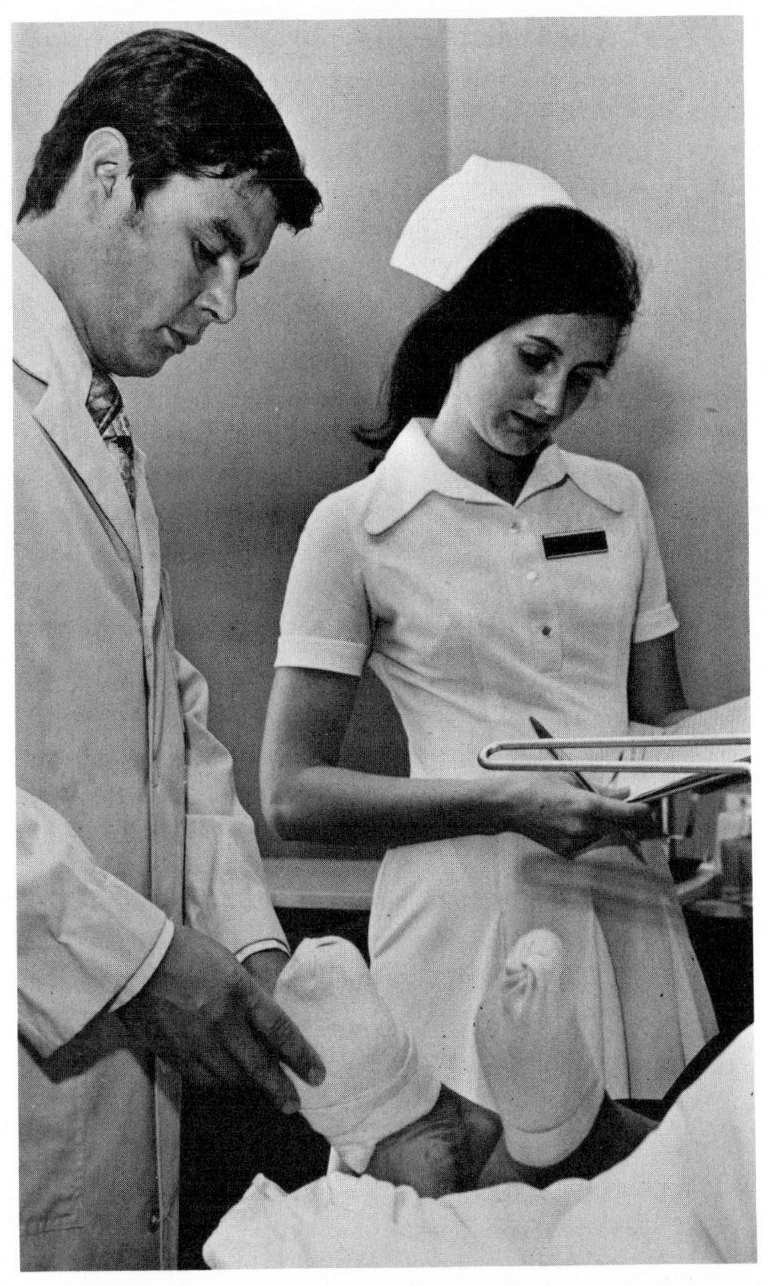

The podiatric surgeon checks the patient on the day following surgery and reviews the vital information assembled by the nurse on his status.

surgery section, he or she is under the complete care of that nurse. She greets him, welcomes him to the OR Suite, allays his fears. This latter function cannot be overvalued as surgery of any kind is an awesome experience for most patients.

Often, they have never had any surgery performed on them before and what is common to any OR personnel could be new and extremely frightening to the patient. William Osler, the great author and surgeon, once said, "The physician will never appreciate the terrible trauma a patient undergoes while in surgery until he himself becomes a patient!"

The OR nurse is usually far more aware of this than the average doctor. She will take a patient who is fearful and cheer him up with her pleasant smile and friendly manner, soft words of encouragement.

In addition to this responsibility, she has the task of making certain that all instruments the surgeon will require are immediately ready and available. Some surgeons have become legendary because of their theatricals, their black moods during surgery. Sometimes they become abusive to those who are assisting them. There is no place in the operating room for a **prima donna.** Any foot surgeon who becomes temperamental or abusive should be immediately censored by his peers. We know of no case where bad manners improved the surgery one whit.

The podiatrist should be understanding when he has difficulty in scheduling a case because of the heavy existing surgical load. The OR Supervisor usually makes sure that the rooms are assigned on a first-come, first-served basis.

Since the OR nurse must scrub for all kinds of surgical cases, she usually has an intimate knowledge of the required instruments and their use. Sometimes a veteran OR nurse will suggest to the podiatrist that he use a different instrument for a given purpose. The wise podiatrist will listen to these suggestions. We know that our own surgery has been improved 100% by the suggestions of friendly and capable OR nurses and they have been a great help in making our current-day surgery sophisticated and oftimes exceptional.

There is no one in the entire hospital that the podiatric surgeon needs more than the OR staff who surround him during his intensive working hours. As with all surgery, there are some great moments, some difficult moments and some very aggravating moments. But there is nothing quite as magnificent in the health picture as the OR team that works hand-in-glove with you to help you in your task and to make you look better through their quiet proficiency and understanding.

The Podiatrist and Medical Records

The medical records of a hospital are a living history of the patient, his hospital stay, laboratory reports concerning his case, treatments rendered and general, overall care. The patient's hospital records constitute a legal document and as such it is important that the podiatrist, like any other physician or surgeon, exercise extreme care in keeping them.

Few physicians or podiatrists are aware that these hospital records must be kept on file for 10 years and they are open to perusal by anyone to whom the patient gives permission to see them.

The important factor in good record keeping is proper documentation. There can be a difference in what the doctor or surgeon actually perform and what is recorded. As far as the hospital records are concerned, if a service is performed for the patient by the physician, but if he fails to document it properly, that service was **not** performed. It is truly imperative that the doctor accurately document every service he performs, otherwise he is exposing both the hospital and himself to a suit, should litigation arise.

Every third year, the Joint Commission on Accreditation of American Hospitals, visits the record room of each hospital to insure that accurate records are being kept and that the medical care is up to standard. Some of the things they look for when inspecting records are a detailed history justifying hospital admission, detailed description of the examination (both medical and podiatric), and a preoperative diagnosis. The operation report must coincide with the entrance diagnosis and the pathological reports.

Every chart must have a complete progress notation and a clinical resume of the patient's hospital stay must also be included. No chart is to be left incomplete for more than 10 days, otherwise the podiatrist and the physician can be subject to suspension of privileges. Finally, keeping the patient's records is the dual responsibility of the physician and the podiatrist.

Some of the common problems encountered by the medical records department usually deal with terminology and improper record keeping. The podiatrist dictating his operation report must remember to speak clearly, slowly and accurately. If he is in doubt as to whether or not the secretary understands him, he should spell the word out. No abbreviations should be used. For example, the abbreviation E.H.L. means nothing to the secretary. The podiatrist must say

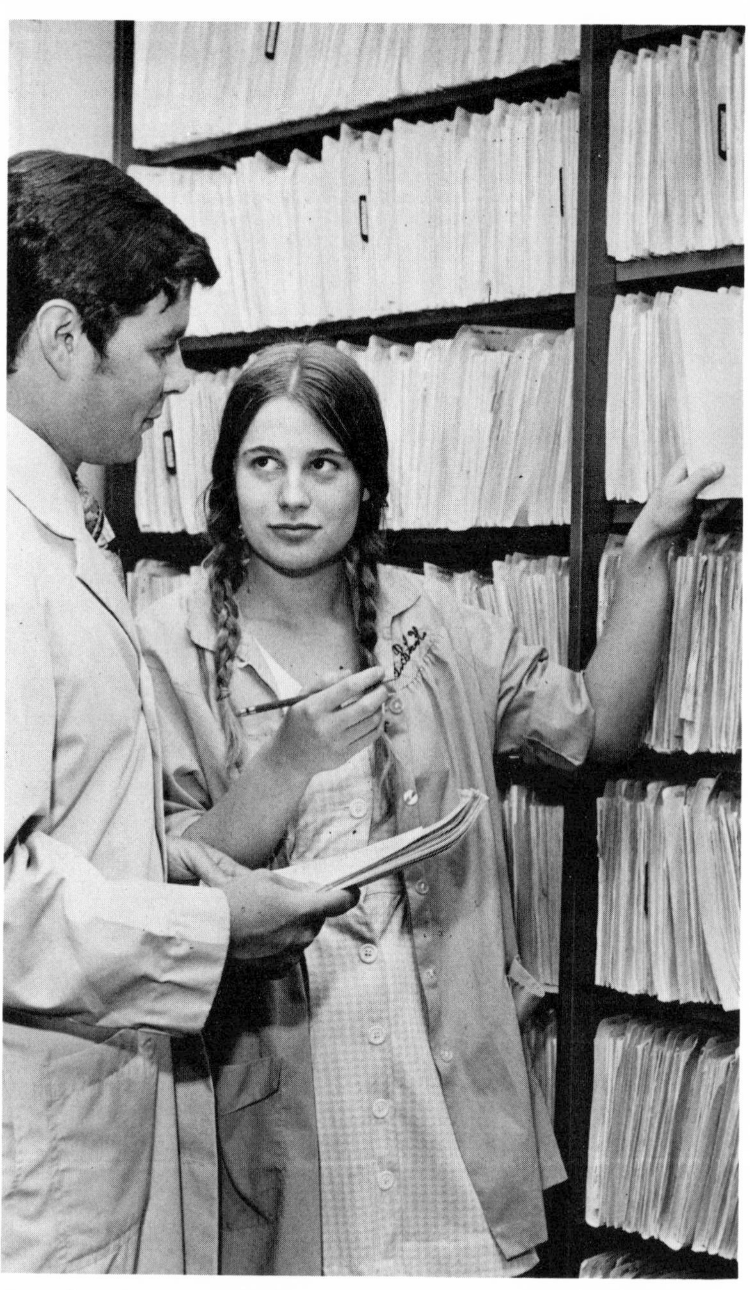

Few physicians or podiatrists are aware that medical records must be kept on file for 10 years.

Extensor Hallucis Longus, to indicate the proper muscle involved.

Another common problem arises in the performance of Osteotripsy techniques (bone rasping techniques). If the surgeon has rasped a bone, he should state that he has performed a resection of bone by rasping. Better to have a little too much explanation than not enough. Often the record department secretaries are confused when they read that a bone has been resected and there is no pathology specimen. Had the surgeon said that he has rasped a bone, she would then understand the reason why no specimen report was included.

In the case of suspected lesions such as Neuromas, the podiatrist usually performs an exploratory and his pre-operative diagnosis may be **possible neuroma**; however, the post-operative diagnosis may prove nerve entrapment or fibro lipoma. It is entirely possible that the pre-operative diagnosis and the post-operative diagnosis will not be the same, which is acceptable as long as an explanation is given. Remember that the doctor cannot say too much in a medical record.

Hospitals that have a podiatric residence program will find that their podiatry records will be excellent because the podiatric resident has more time to complete his records. However, there are two pitfalls that often occur which the wise podiatrist will avoid. One is that the staff podiatrist will get spoiled and very often not have any progress notes written by himself since he is permitting the residents to do this work. The result will be a chart which has his name on the Operation Report and nowhere else, almost as though he were a ghost. The podiatrist should make an effort to personally write a progress report on the patient's hospital stay at least every other day.

The second pitfall is more serious. Sometimes the resident will become so used to writing progress notes that, after awhile, he will begin to dictatorialize in his notes. Sometimes the resident may not agree with the attending surgeon's choice of techniques and he might put down in the progress notes that the technique was unnecessary or unwise. This kind of editorializing must be censored immediately, since it can only lead to future problems. This is not to say that the resident is not permitted to express his feelings but that he should do so in person and not on the record.

All of the above which is true in the record room applies equally to nearly every other phase of the podiatrist's activities within the hospital realm. The podiatrist who is meticulous and has a conscience will not fail to observe the basic rules in all his hospital activities. He will brief the co-admitting physician so that he understands what the podiatric problems of the patient are, he will plainly inform the nurse, who may not have handled this kind of patient before what he wishes done for the patient, he will point out to the radiologist what he is looking for in the patient's foot x-rays, he will be as specific in the pathological or clinical laboratory.

The podiatrist who establishes or goes to work in a hospital podiatry section enters a strange world to which he must accustom himself. He must become familiar with the mores and traditions of the hospital staff and respect them and, if he does, he himself will find acceptance in time. In the same fashion, his specialty and techniques and needs are unfamiliar to the hospital technicians and staff. If he takes the time to teach them the rudiments of what is required of them, everyone will benefit.

Podiatric Advances in Recent Years —The New Techniques

In tracing the history of podiatry through the first half of our century, we become aware that while podiatrists made some substantial advances during these years, they were principally of a non-surgical nature. When operative techniques did start improving, the innovations came with a rush.

Perhaps the father of modern foot surgery, as we have come to know it today, is Dr. Earl G. Kaplan, of Detroit, Michigan. In 1956, this progressive podiatrist organized a group in Detroit, which created the Civic Hospital of Detroit, an institution devoted entirely to podiatric surgery and treatment.

In this hospital, with its aggressive and progressive staff, Dr. Kaplan inaugurated the first truly surgical residency in podiatry and trained scores of capable practitioners who migrated to all parts of the nation bringing his updated surgical gospel with them.

In addition to training residents, Civic Hospital inaugurated weekend surgical programs for practitioners from various parts of the country, to teach them the basics of foot surgery. This was not an easy task since textbooks on the subject were virtually non-existent. Many of the standard procedures used in foot surgery today were begun here.

The 60's opened up many new horizons for the podiatrist, with his acceptance by national health insurance companies, Medicare and Medicaid. In this decade, too, the now-famous Bulletin #44, published by the Joint Commission on the Accreditation of American Hospitals, gave hospital podiatry the opportunity to be born, to grow and to prosper.

The 1970's started off most auspiciously with a greater growth and refinement of podiatric surgery than had occurred in all the years preceding it. With the '70's also came new residency programs in podiatric surgery in hospitals throughout the country. Aid from the Federal Government for podiatric students considerably increased the enrollment in the podiatric colleges, whose existing facilities then had to be enlarged. With Federal recognition and aid, there evolved a mass of highly qualified students who demanded and got a finer and more substantial education than had podiatrists in the past.

The programs that were new in the late '60's matured in the early '70's and many refinements and advances in technical achievement over previous years were inaugurated. For example, the availability of new, sophisticated, modern power equipment and excellent surgical facilities caused the field of adductory wedging, osteotomies, fusions and a host of other intricate bone surgeries to become common practice among podiatric surgeons.

Some techniques which were written years ago, but were not deemed practical because of the lack of proper equipment, were now put into use and improved. For example, the Reverdin procedure for Hallux Valgus was first written 92 years ago. However, with the finer equipment and facilities, it has become an accepted and standard procedure among working podiatrists.

The same can be said of the Lapidus and Meisenbach procedures. These also are not new in origin but have been revised and put into accepted use. In the case of Lapidus, it has become a practical procedure for the correction of Metatarsus Primus Varus. In the case of the Meisenbach procedure, it has been revised under the name of Osteoclasis, which is an extremely popular procedure today for the elevation of a Planti-flexed Metatarsal shaft.

The modern podiatric surgeon has become both imaginative and prolific in introducing new techniques and it will probably be some years before the written literature catches up with him.

There was a statement made some years ago that podiatry was a parasitic profession insofar as medical literature was concerned. This was fairly true, podiatry had virtually no literature. This does not imply that the podiatrist lacked the material or the talent to create authoritative and creative texts in his specialty. As the profession improved, as new advances were made, the podiatrist did start recording his achievements. Certainly the work of Dr. Philip Brachman in the late '30's and '40's, with his ambulatory reciprocal bar for the correction of inward and outward gait problems, has benefited the entire medical profession. There have been many others as well.

Marvin Steinberg, D.P.M., of New York, has long been a leading light of podiatric medicine and pathology. He has created not only unique medications but has also become the father of a dermatological entity, Poro Keratosis Discreta, a common lesion found in the foot, which is caused by the plugging up of the sweat glands.

Another reason for the lack of podiatric literature was that the established medical publishers did not wish to publish podiatric books. They felt that the market was too small and uncertain for them to make a profit. They also felt that only a qualified medical doctor could be authoritative, even in the field of podiatry.

However, the worm has turned. The startling success of recent podiatric books, written and published by podiatrists, themselves, have been so great that now the medical publishers are keenly interested in publishing literature for the profession.

In the years to come, we will see many fine books, authored by knowledgeable podiatrists, concerning all aspects of podiatric medicine on the shelves of libraries all over the nation. There are podiatrists who are capable and competent but who have no flair for translating their technical accomplishments into the written word. But there are many others, with a deep love for writing and teaching, who will take up the gauntlet and produce a bank of literature on the subject of podiatry that will be second to none.

The future is certainly wide open to all manner of new developments and techniques in the field of podiatric medicine. To mention one thought that comes to mind, the field of implant surgery has grown so rapidly that one can foresee the replacement of total bone segments such as Metatarsal Shafts, Cuboids and even the Calcaneus.

Recent simian surgery carried out by podiatrists may one day lead to the transplantation of a viable foot. How is that for practical dreaming? But you can believe it and you can also believe that no other field is as wide open to progress and invention as the podiatric profession. The horizons are limitless, the future resplendent with promise of new achievements and fortune awaits every ambitious and creative podiatrist in this great and rewarding profession.

Reverdin Operation

The Reverdin Operation is an old technique which has been revived in podiatric surgery. It aims at the correction of Hallux Valgus by realigning the lateral, displaced articular facet of the first metatarsal. This is accomplished by a wedge ostectomy.

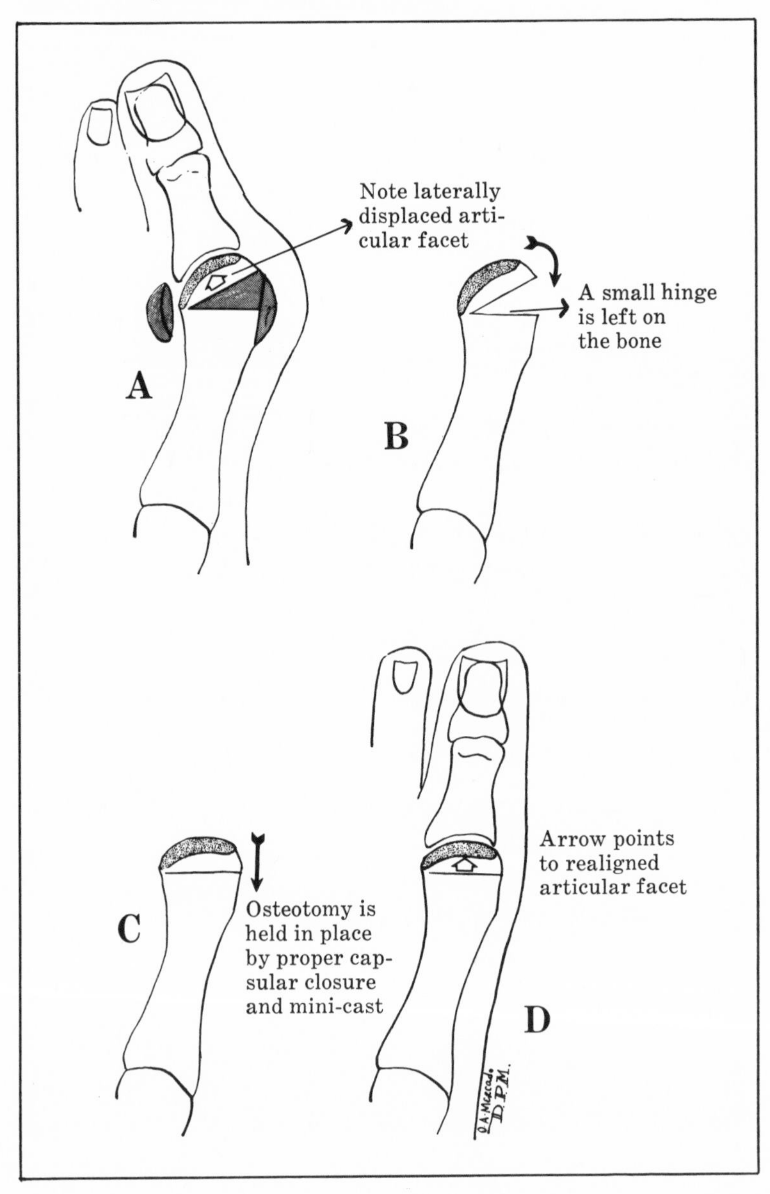

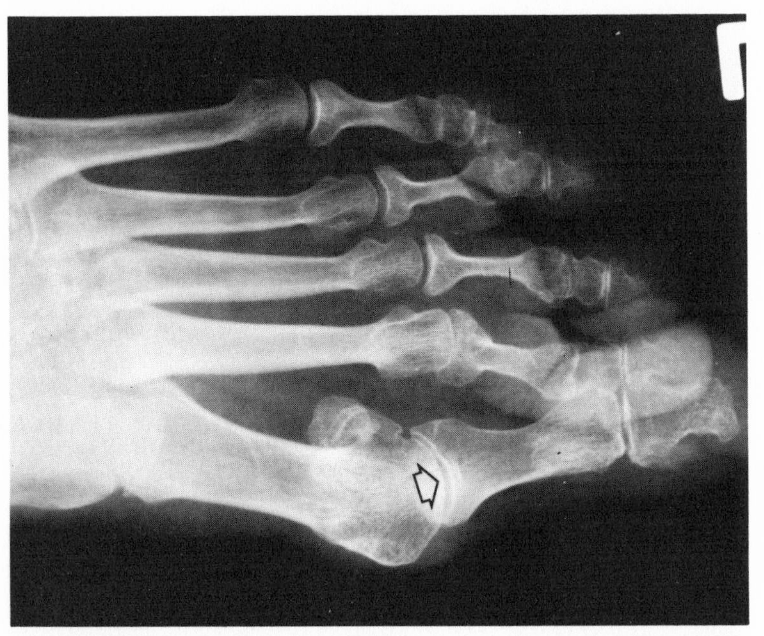

Before

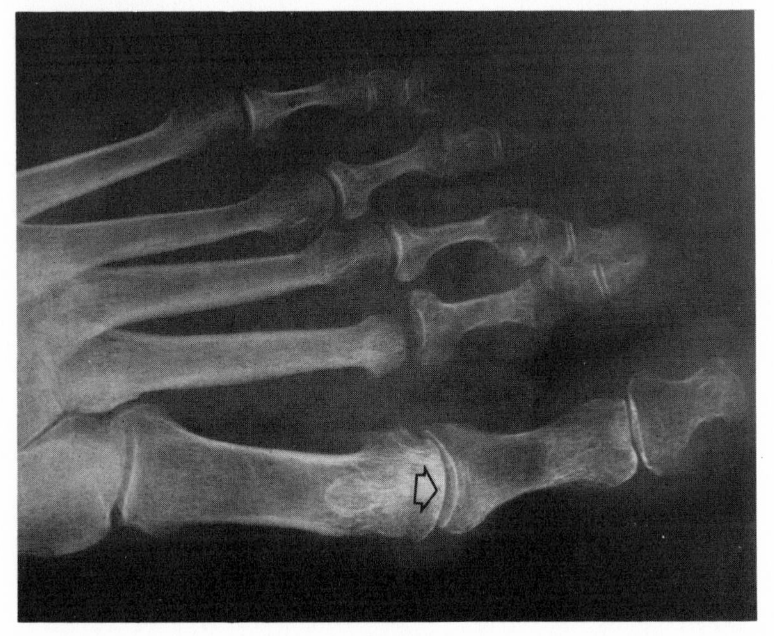

After

The Lapidus Operation

The Lapidus Operation is another old technique which podiatric surgeons have modified and improved upon. It aims at the correction of metatarsus primus varus by the fusion of the first metatarsal cuneiform articulation.

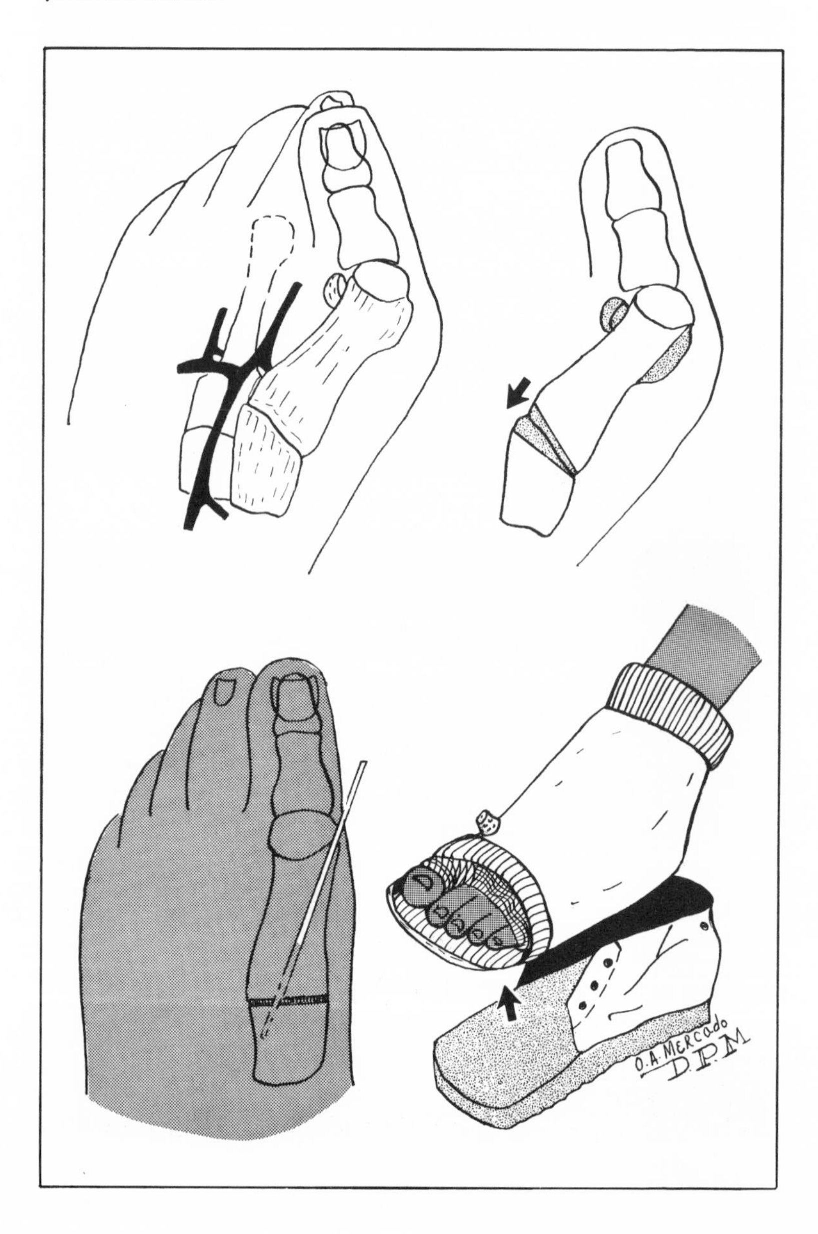

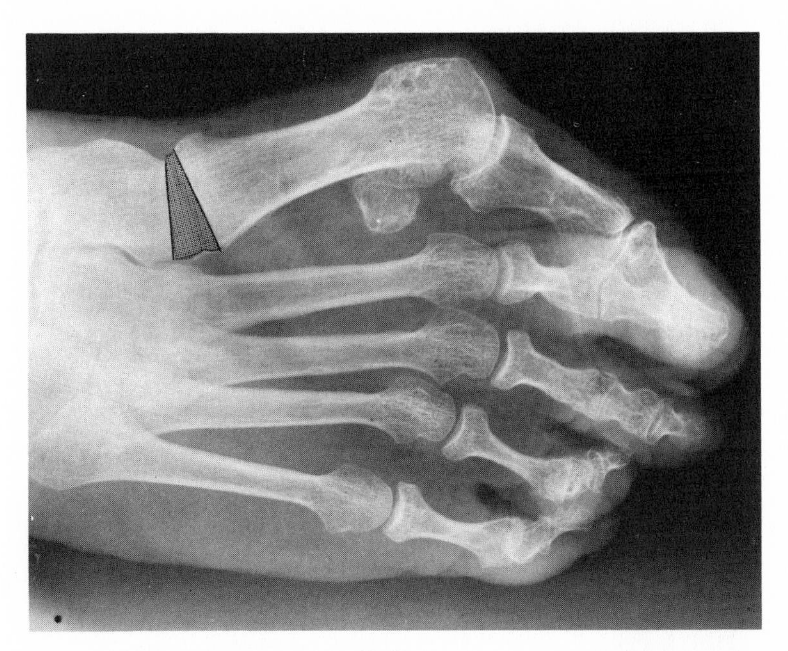

Before

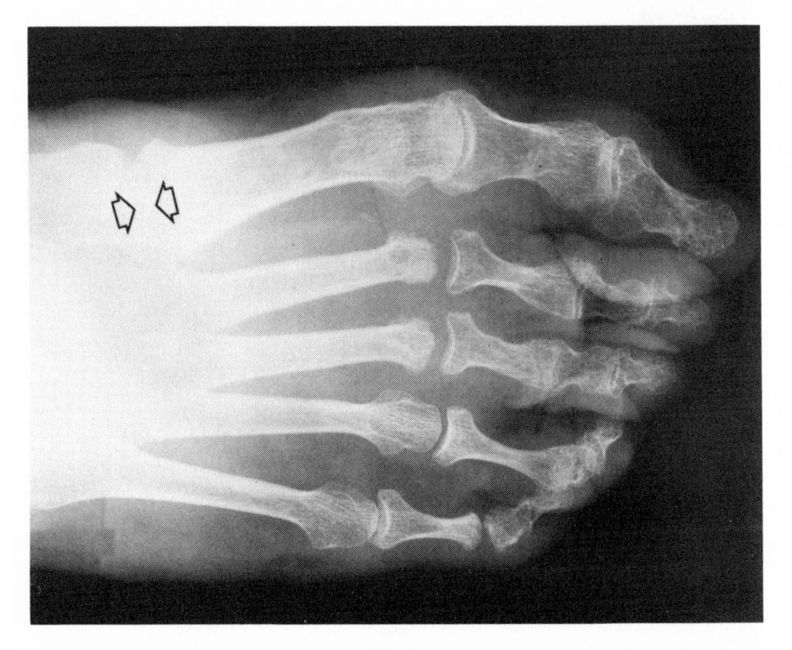

After

Technique for Silastic Implant

The field of joint replacements by silastic implants has burgeoned in recent years and the podiatrist has contributed greatly to the perfection of this technique.

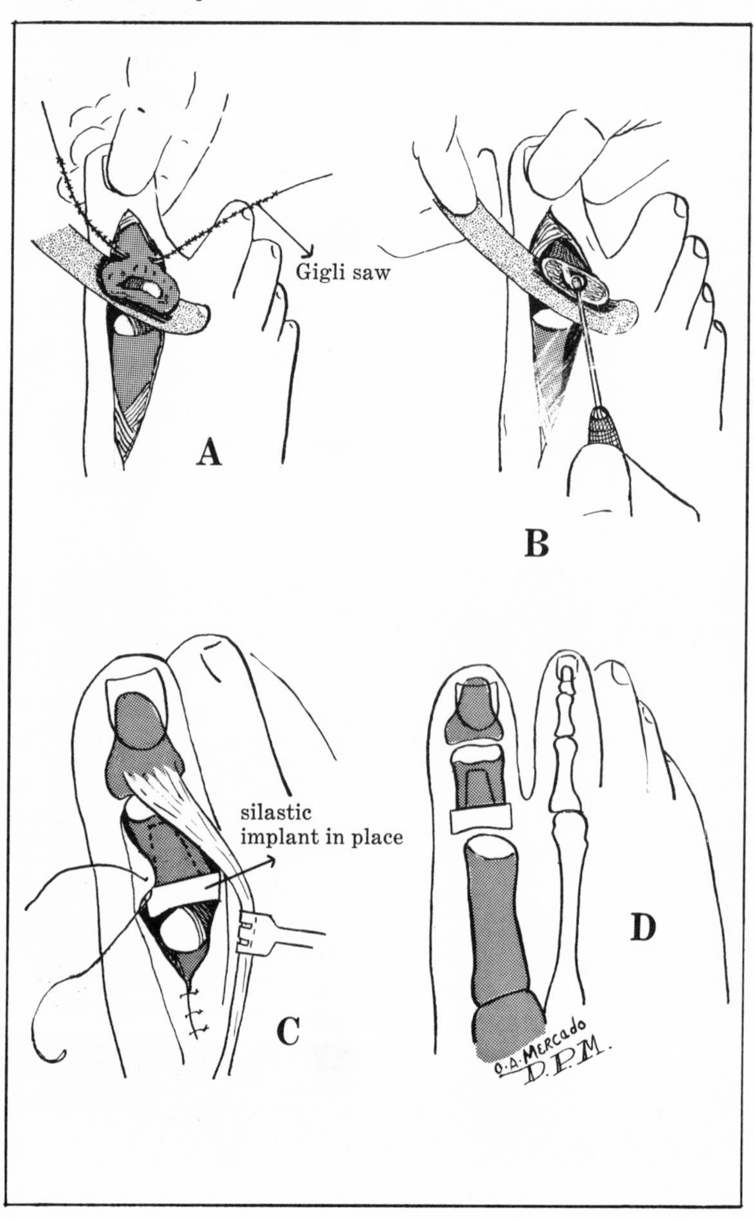

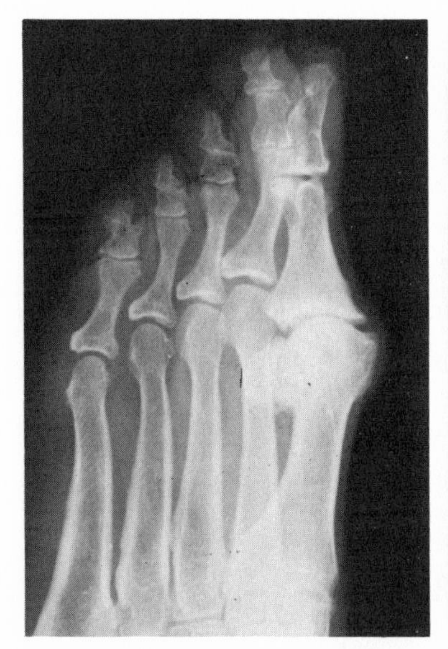
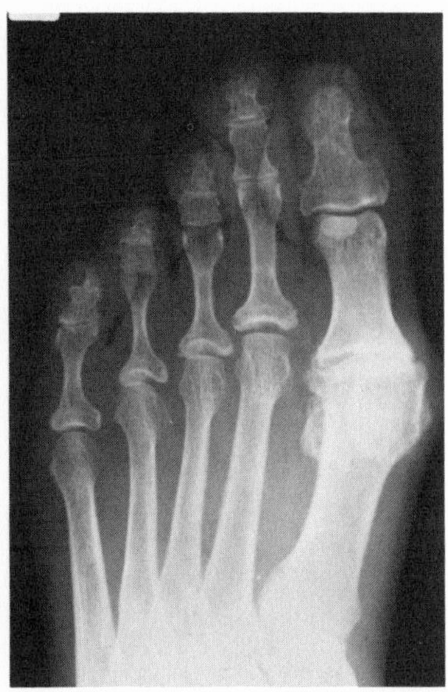

Here is an arthritic joint (First Metatarsal Phalangeal Joint)

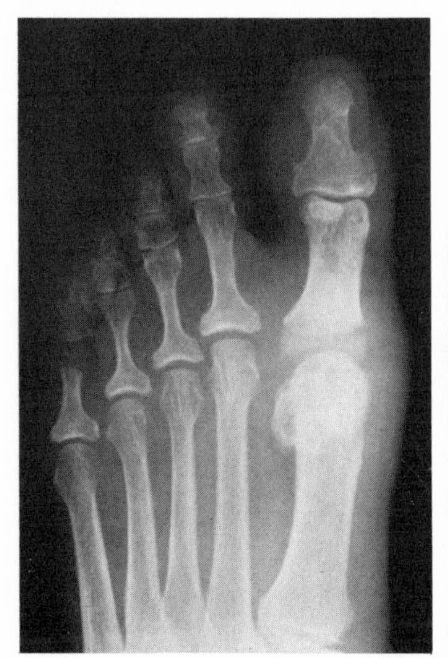
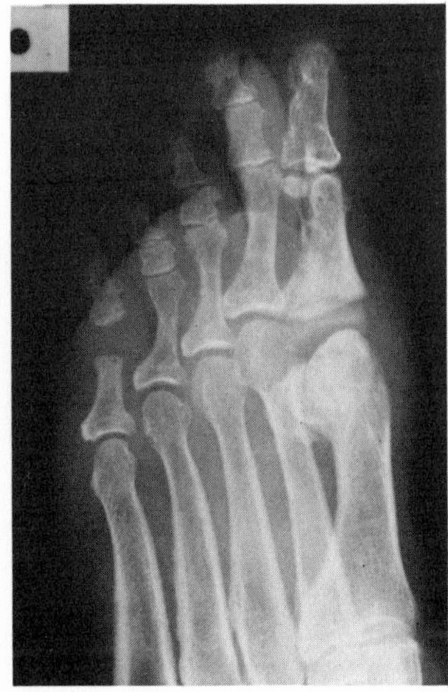

repaired with the use of silastic insert.

McKeever Operation

A technique used to shorten elongated lesser metatarsal rays and is ideally suited for a Morton's type Syndrome where the elongated second metatarsal ray has caused an intractable planter keratosis (I.P.K.)

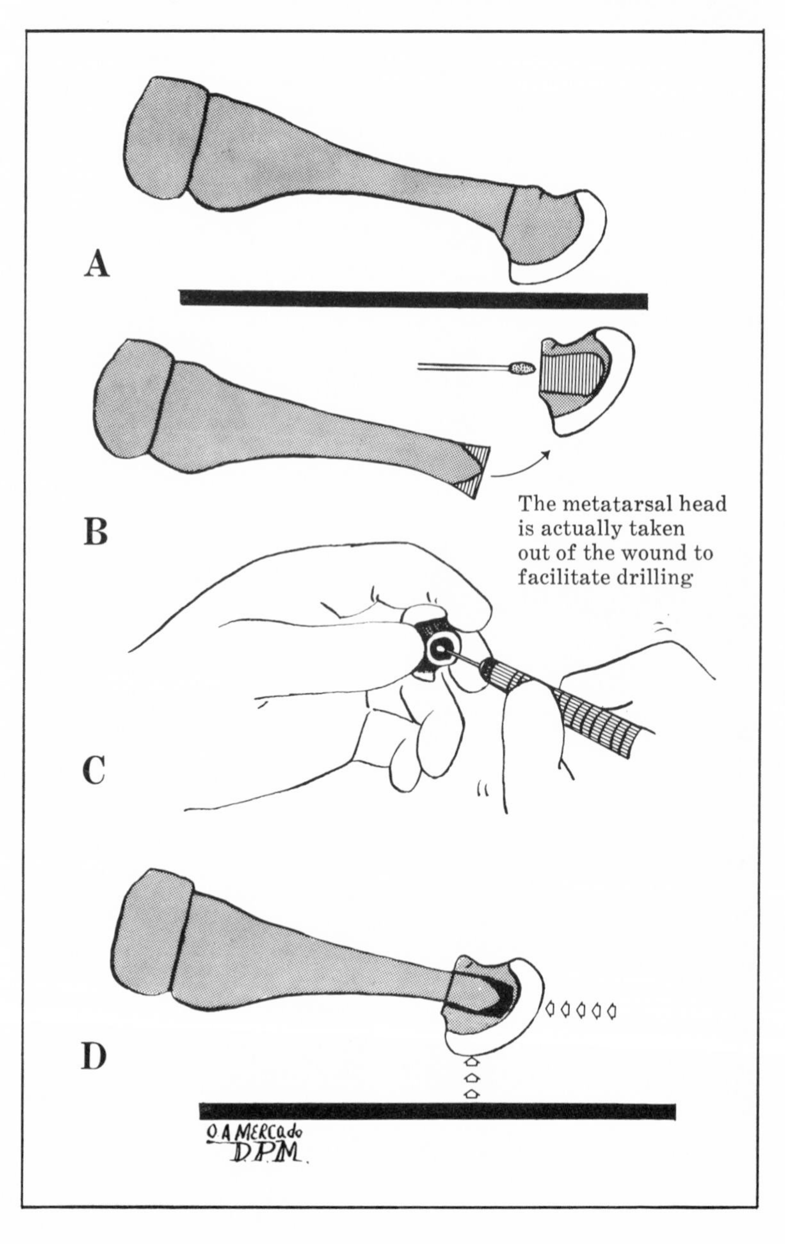

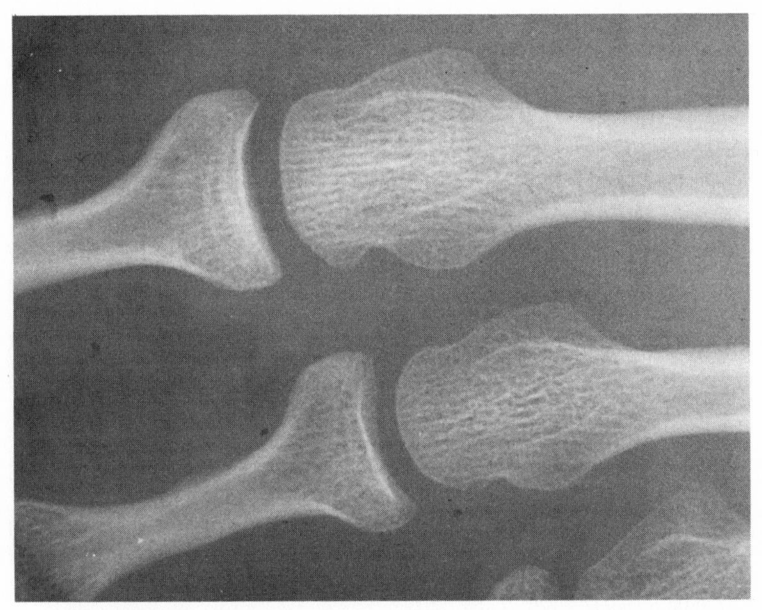

Pre-operative x-ray of elongated second metatarsal ray.

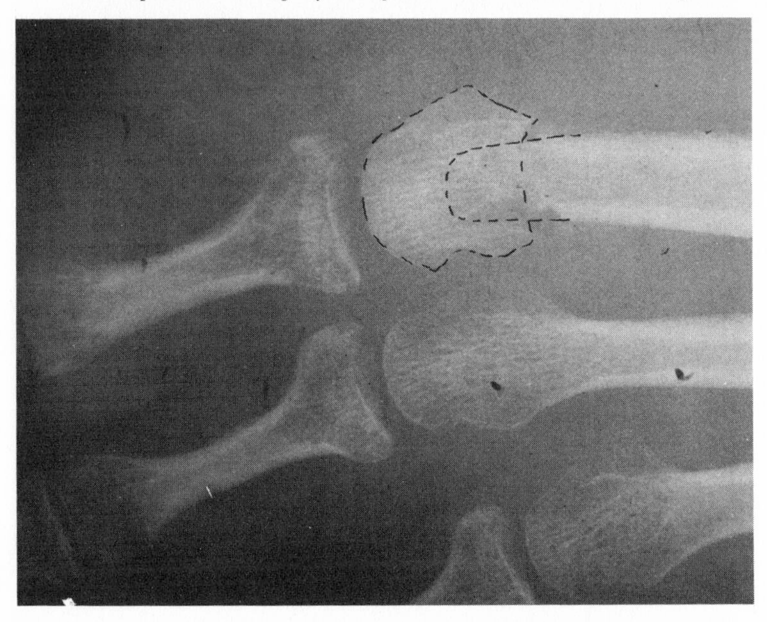

Three weeks post-operative x-ray of McKeever operation. Dotted line shows reamed out head fitting over truncated metatarsal shaft.

Heel Spur Osteotripsy

The heel spur osteotripsy (bone rasping) was developed in podiatric surgery for the surgical treatment of heel spurs.

Figure A shows the proper placement of the foot when a radiograph is taken; Figure B the hyperostotic shelving (heel spur) of the calcaneal tuberosities is shown; Figure C after the area has been properly masked, a rasp is introduced and the spur is reduced. This simplified technique reduces the post-operative recuperation period of the patient.

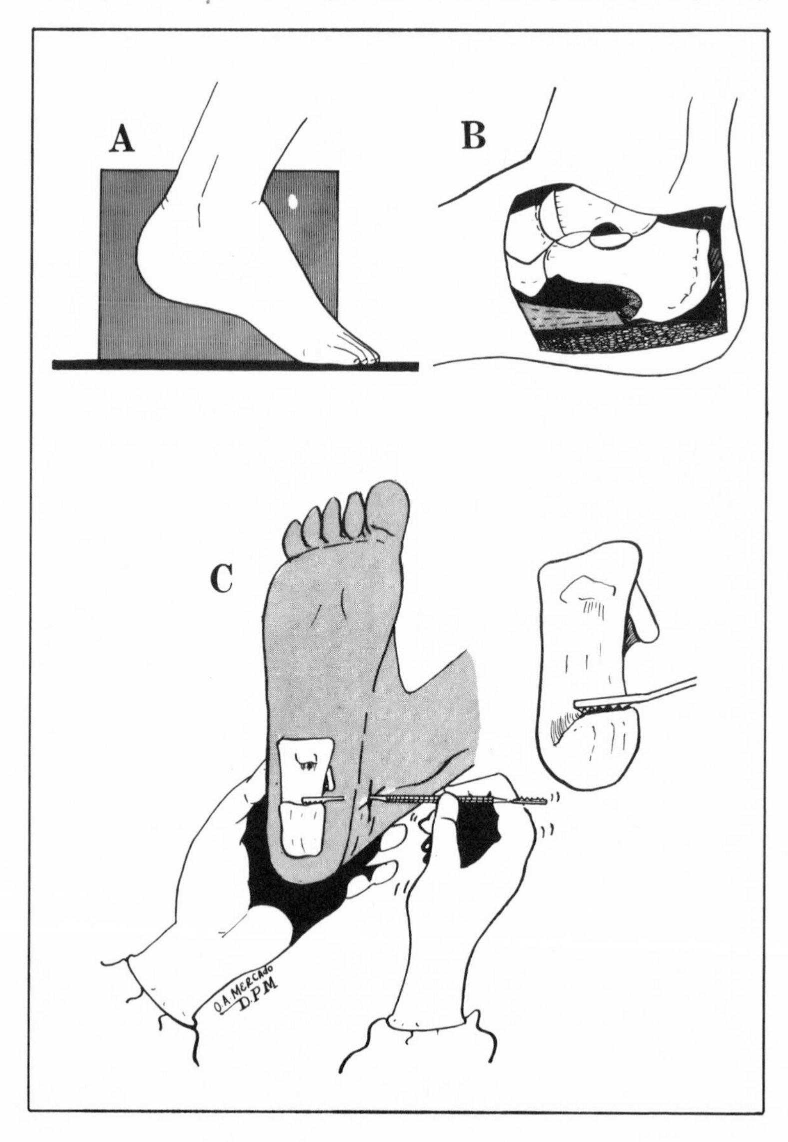

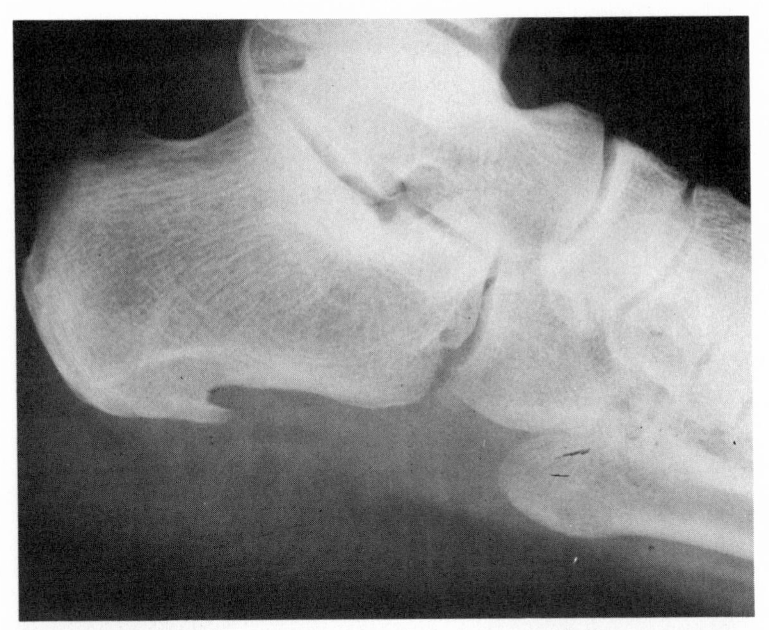

The top figure shows a pre-operative view of a typical heel spur.

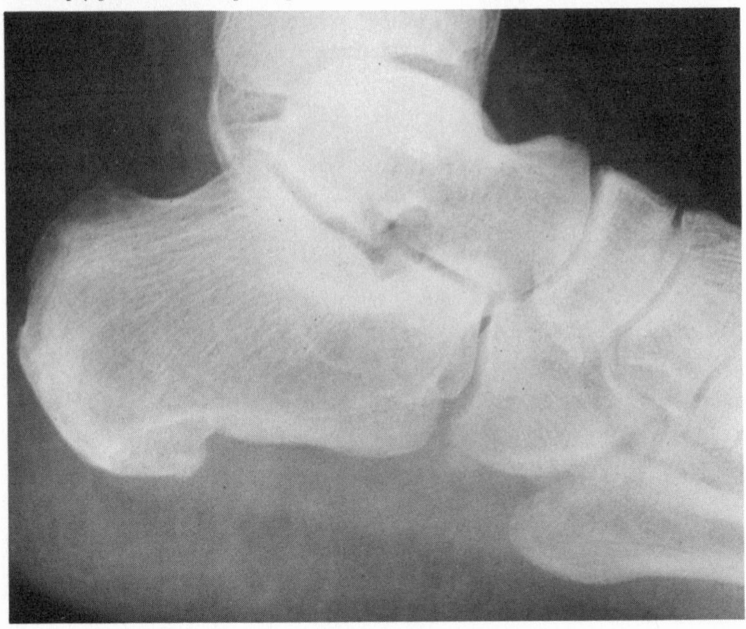

The bottom figure shows a post-operative view. The heel spur is reduced by osteotripsy (bone rasping) techniques.

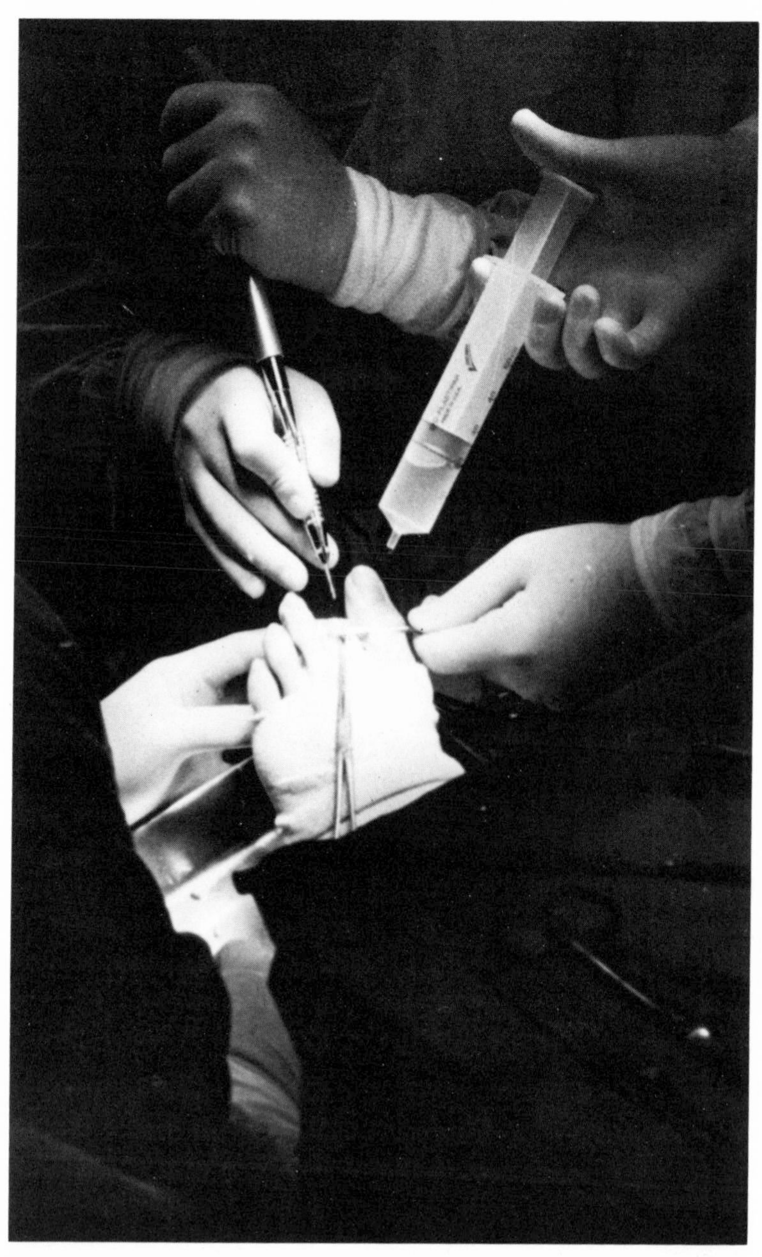

Modern techniques and instruments permit the podiatric surgeon to excel in his specialty. Here a small joint is being replaced with a silastic insert.

Podiatric Hospital Residencies

There are 47 institutions throughout the country today offering 151 positions for postgraduate training in podiatric surgery. These include colleges, hospitals, state and rehabilitation institutions. The graduating D.P.M. now has available to him, 111 first-year residency programs, 14 second-year residency programs and one third-year program.

There are also 25 training programs which have received provisional approval by the Council On Podiatry Education of the American Podiatry Association. This Council has the task of inspecting and accrediting all postgraduate training programs in podiatry which request evaluation of their particular educational activities.

The growth of podiatric residency programs in this decade has been phenomenal. Today, approximately one-third of all graduating D.P.M.'s will have a good chance of obtaining an accredited residency program that will prepare them to meet the challenge of modern podiatry. It is estimated that in the next two or three years, there will be enough programs available for every graduating D.P.M. who desires postgraduate training, to obtain it.

Why has the growth of podiatric residencies been so great in the past few years? Some of the experts feel that there is an instrinsic motivating growth force in all podiatric residency programs. Dr. E. Dalton McGlamry, President of the American Podiatry Association and chairman of the podiatry section of Doctor's Hospital in Tucker, Georgia, feels that the presence of podiatric residents in any hospital podiatry section, will provide better patient care, afford them the opportunity of learning more sophisticated surgical techniques and keep the attending podiatry staff on their toes and up-to-date on the latest techniques, which they must impart to the younger residents.

The one-year training program is usually a rotating type of program, consisting of a succession of weeks in pathology, anesthesia, radiology and surgery. The junior or one-year resident will also spend much of his time attending podiatry clinical conferences and lectures by members of the medical and podiatry staffs. In some institutions, they are also expected to spend part of their time in research and writing.

At the end of the one-year period, these residents will have acquired practical knowledge in record keeping, pre- and post-op care of patients, emergency care, clinical medicine, and surgical dexterity. They will have also acquired a good didactic background in all aspects of medicine and surgery. In our hospital the first-year junior residents spend every other afternoon with the chief of medical education, Milton Miller, M.D. The residents accompany Dr. Miller on his medical rounds, and they learn the art of history taking and physical diagnosis. This includes ausculation of the heart and lungs and even the examination of the fundi.

The second-year residency concerns itself mostly with the actual practice of podiatric surgery. The senior resident has the responsibility of making assignments for the junior residents and students. Along with a staff member, he is the discussant at all clinical podiatry conferences. He is expected to spend a good deal of time in anesthesia and clinical research. Actually, in our hospital, six months of the second year are spent in anesthesia, under the tutelage of Fern Sanner, M.D., Chief of Anesthesia Services. Here they learn emergency management, intubation, the art of general anesthesia as well as local and perfusion anesthesia.

When we first introduced the program for anesthesia to our residency program, there was a lot of flack from some of the podiatrists. They felt that, perhaps, we were losing track of our goal which is to train fully-qualified foot surgeons. However, we felt that anesthesia and emergencies are part and parcel of any surgeon's training. The men who have taken and completed our course, far from being "pseudo M.D.'s" are fully competent foot surgeons who are aware of their limitations and confident of their knowledge. It is hoped that the other residency

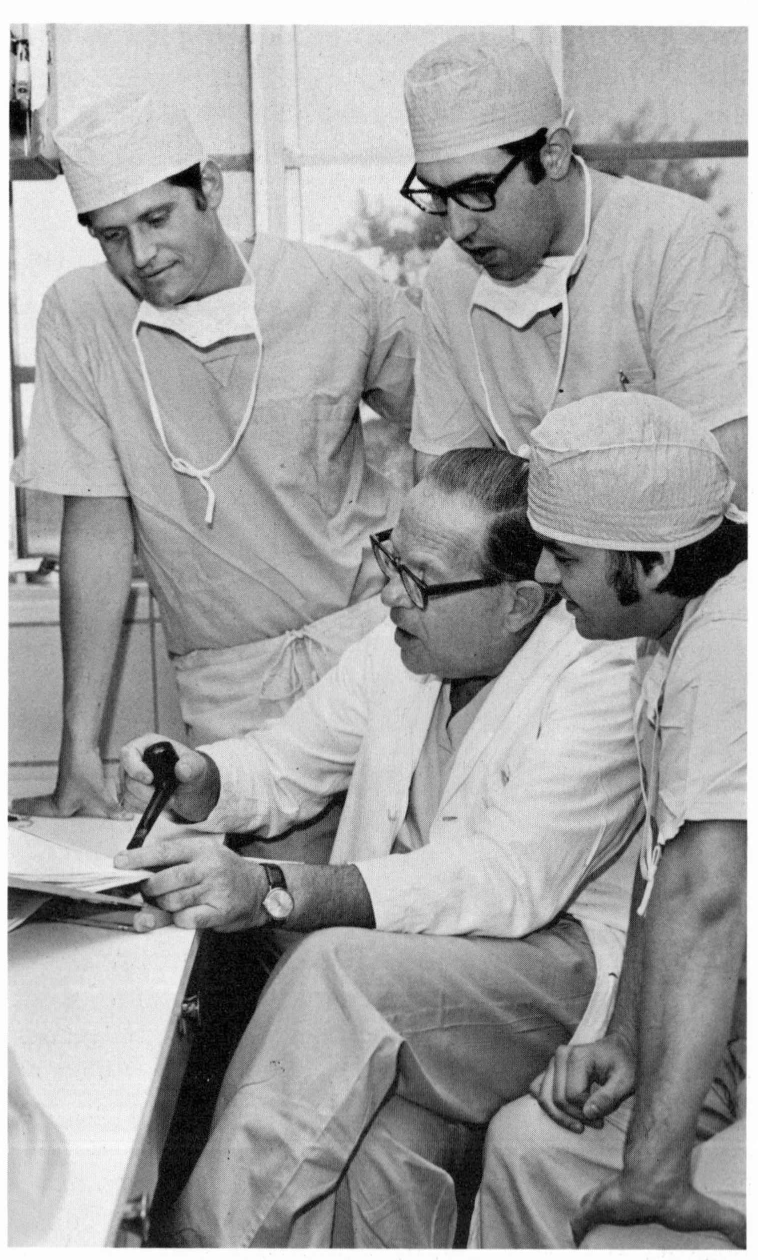

A general surgeon reviews a case with some podiatry residents at a hospital. His advice on occasionally difficult or perplexing cases can often be beyond price.

programs throughout the country will adopt as vigorous a training in anesthesia as we have.

There is only one third-year residency training program at the present time. This program is at Doctor's Hospital in Tucker, Georgia, and is conducted by E. Dalton McGlamry, D.P.M. Doctor's Hospital is an osteopathic hospital of 238 beds and is considered one of the finest with one of the best residency programs in the country.

The prerequisites for obtaining admission to the three-year program is to have completed a two-year residency in an accredited institution. The graduate of the Doctor's Hospital three-year residency program is a far cry indeed from the itinerant corn cutter of yesteryear.

THE PODIATRIC RESIDENT

The podiatric resident is no different than any other resident in any specialty of medicine. He is usually young, aggressive, ambitious and, certainly, to have graduated from any present-day health institution, quite intelligent. In other words, he is a man of excellent caliber and promise.

In medicine, the youthful graduate has his choice of hospitals where he can serve his internship and where the salary is excellent. In podiatry, since there are three graduates to every program available, at this writing, the competition to get into one of these programs is fast and furious. The stipend for this program is, as a rule, below par and often inadequate. But the truth of the matter is the old law of supply and demand and the youthful podiatrist should recognize the facts and not be discouraged.

A few short years ago, the chance of any graduating D.P.M. getting a residency program was completely dismal. The American Podiatry Association is meeting the challenge of creating more good podiatric residencies head-on and their success has been truly sensational. By the time this volume is printed, there will probably be a 20% increase in residency programs; they are growing fast. We can emphatically predict that the class starting podiatry school this year will have more residencies available to them than they will need when they graduate.

The first objective of the American Podiatry Association has been to create programs. Their next objective will be to bring all programs up to a level of quality that is acceptable to themselves and to the medical profession as well. While the graduate of yesteryear had to put up with inadequate training, the future graduate will be obtaining a postgraduate training and education equal to that of any other medical specialist.

The podiatric resident has the responsibility to the staff, the hospital, the profession and the patient to always do his best. Often there have been problems with the over-zealous resident who has attempted to do things beyond his abilities. He must remember that everything he does, good or bad, reflects directly on the podiatric staff in particular and on the profession in general. The podiatric resident should remember that, if he has any questions or problems, he should clear them through the Chief of the Podiatry Service. To try to go over the head of the departmental chief is a grievous error.

There is an inherent problem with most residents, whether they be podiatric or medical, which is that as he acquires knowledge, he begins to feel the need to express himself. William Nolan, in his best-selling book, "The Making of a Surgeon", states that surgery by nature is a very egotistical field. At one point in his training, a surgeon-to-be feels that he is capable of handling any surgical program in his specialty as well or better than anyone else.

The need to express himself often comes to the surface in the form of criticism by the podiatrist of the training program. Stuart M. Ruch, D.P.M. of Pekin, Illinois, one of the founders of the Hopedale Medical Complex residency program, states that one of the major problems encountered by podiatric residents is that they feel they just aren't performing enough surgery.

Many podiatric residents enter upon their training with the erroneous idea that their primary business is to operate. Frederick F. Boyce, M.D. of Tulane University School of Medicine, Department of Surgery, writes on the surgical resident, saying that "while the surgical resident will spend much of his time in the Operating Room . . . the basis of the residency system is one of progressive delegation of responsibility, including the responsibility of operating, but permission to operate is always a late privilege, not an early one—and justifiably so.

The resident must be closely supervised for many weary hours (they are much more weary for his preceptor), before he is permitted to stand alone in the Operating Room. There is nothing worse for a young surgeon than too much freedom when he is just beginning to learn the many facets of his specialty."

Dr. Ruch brings forth another important problem which is that the residents often feel they know more than the attending staff. Comment on this point is almost unnecessary. A humble attitude will stand the beginner in very good stead while he is learning the many fine points of the difficult and often complex surgical aspects of his podiatric education.

Too often, the resident, in his youthful exuberance, forgets that the reason he is in a program is because podiatrists before him worked hard and long to better the profession and create the opportunity. It cannot be stated too strongly that every podiatric resident is his brother's keeper and he should act accordingly.

What Tomorrow Holds for the Hospital Podiatrist

We have traced the growth of podiatry from the times of the itinerant corn cutter to the experienced and highly qualified modern-day foot surgeon. A whole world separates these two men—a world of difference in training, background, technical abilities and in their basic concept of the profession. Comparing the two men and their respective talents is like comparing the old frontier's horse-and-buggy doctor with the sophisticated surgical specialist of today.

There are those in the profession who feel that podiatry is now a far cry from the career they went into years ago. They are right. No one, not even the most optimistic professionals could have foreseen the tremendous thrusts forward made by podiatry, especially in the field of surgery.

What was once rightfully known as chiropody is no more. Podiatrists are no longer a group of itinerant corn cutters but proven experts in a medical specialty which they have nurtured and developed into a highly respectable and challenging profession.

Where do we go from here? What challenges must future podiatrists meet? Are we destined to become absorbed by medicine and so lose our identity or will we continue to grow and prosper as an individual specialty in the medical arena?

In a recent editorial, Dr. E. Dalton McGlamry, president of the American Podiatry Association, warned that we must not lose track of podiatry in our somewhat frenzied quest for medical acceptance. To provide the basic podiatric care which has been responsible for the growth of our profession is fully as important as our phenomenal growth and competence in the field of surgery.

There are those who are unequivocally opposed to this kind of thinking. They believe that growth is an accepted fact in our changing society and if we wish to avoid "future shock" as a profession, we must accept the fact that podiatry, as we knew it, no longer exists. They feel that podiatry has become a part of medicine and we should push with all our efforts and energies to become assimilated by the medical profession.

This group of podiatrists give credence to the argument that there are forces within the medical profession which are crying for a change. They want to see medicine become more people-oriented; in other words, they are pressing for accelerated medical schools and merging of basic science instruction, so that health professionals can all attend two years of basic sciences and from there go into a specialty, whether it be general practice, general surgery, eye surgery, oral surgery or foot surgery.

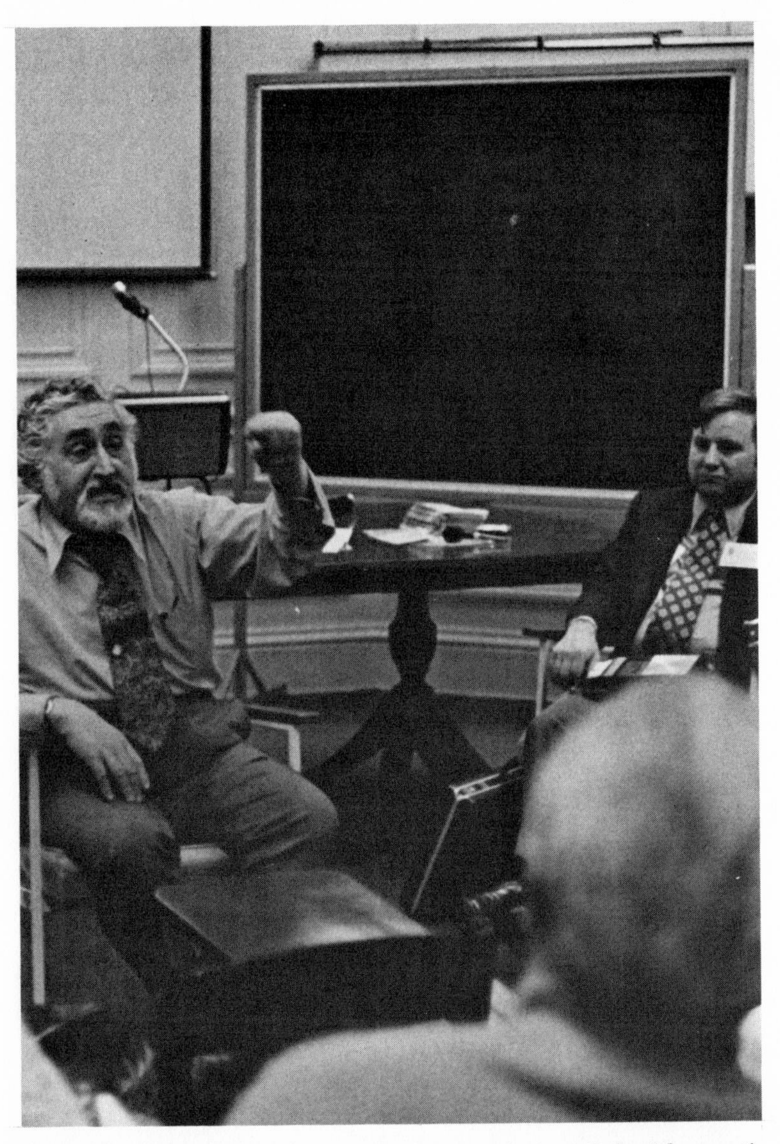

Postgraduate training is becoming a "must" for all health practitioners. Here, in a workshop, problem medical cases are discussed.

Our feeling is that there is truth and substance to both arguments. But, in a sense, we tend to agree with Dr. McGlamry. Podiatrists must never forget that the "raison d'etre" of podiatry is to provide needed foot care for the public. The podiatrist practicing in the large urban centers will find that, if he so desires, he can specialize in one field, such as surgery. The podiatrist in the small community will find that he has a responsibility to the public to provide overall foot care. Each must meet and accept his own destiny, the one that makes him happiest, provides the best care for his patients and the best living for himself and his family.

Of course, these are random thoughts, it could all go in another direction. But this much we know. The growth of podiatry and the innovation of the hospital podiatry section will continue in expansion and importance and in the number of programs set up throughout the country. Because of the importance of the service provided by the hospital podiatrist, he will eventually emerge as a full equal to any other member of the medical staff and his influence in the hospital team will be substantial.

With the influx of new residency training programs, the hospitals will have great numbers of competent men to choose from. As more and more of these men are accepted into the hospital scene, and prove their worth, the new image of the podiatrist will replace that which has been held for so many years by members of the medical staff. A new respect and a new comradeship will develop which will reflect well on the podiatrist and mark his continuing progress in the field.

Professions are like children, they have growing

problems. Podiatry is going through such a phase today. When it was chiropody in the early years, it got little respect and, in truth, deserved little. Who was to foresee that this "sideline" would develop into the solid, imaginative, creative and demanding profession it has become today? Who could know that from no formal schooling at all, it would progress to the point where the requirements would be as formidable as those required of any other medical specialist?

We have a precious thing in our hands. We should manipulate it wisely, protect its good name, gain the respect of our peers, obtain the recognition and approval of the public and project the dignity and prestige we possess as practitioners of a fine and worthwhile profession.

BIBLIOGRAPHY

A Manual of Hospital Podiatry

Blauch, Lloyd E.: 1964 Survey of the Podiatry Profession—Podiatry Services and Practices: J.A.P.A. Vol. 8, Aug. 1965.

Blauch, Lloyd E.: et. al.: The Podiatry Curriculum. AM. Assoc. Coll. Pod. Med. 1970, Washington, D.C.

Conwell, Donald P.: Community Podiatry, A Challenge for the Seventies. J.A.P.A. Col. 59, Jan. 1969.

Conwell, Donald P.: Community Podiatry—One Year After. J.A.P.A. Vol. 59, Nov. 1969.

DeMoon, Patrick A.: Editorial, Hosp. Podiatry Review Vol. 1, Spring Issue 1973.

DeMoon, Patrick A.: Editorial, Hosp. Podiatry Review Vol. 1, Fall Issue 1973.

Dorothy, W. L. et al.: The Role of Podiatry N. Engl. J. Med. 284 - 24 June, 1971.

Greenfield, H. I.: Manpower Supply and New Health Delivery System. Bull. N.Y. Acad. Med. 47 ,Sept. 1971.

Helfand, Arthur E.: Practical Guide for Podiatric Programs in Extended Care Facilities. A.P.A. Vol. 56, May 1966.

Helms, D. C.: Podiatry, A Needed Dimension in Medical Care. N. Eng. J. Med, 284 - 18 Mar. 1971.

Horowitz, H.; Luper, T.; and Prezioss, I.: A Podiatry Out-Patient Department in a General Hospital. J.A.P.A. Vol. 53, No. 7, 1963.

Joint Commission on Accreditation of Hospitals: Accreditation Manual of Hospitals 1970, Chicago, Illinois.

Joint Commission Standards Governing Hospital Privileges for Podiatrists. Wisc. Med. J. 67, Jan. 1968.

Kane, John M.: Podiatry Within a State Hospital. J.A.P.A. Vol. 56, Nov. 1966.

Kirschner, Carl; Bartis, Joseph R.; Denno, Gordon: In Hospital Training for Podiatrists. J.A.P.A. Vol. 53, July 1963.

Klein, Berts: Implications of Intermediaries in Podiatry. J.A.P.A. Vol. 59, Sept. 1969.

Macken, Owen: Setting a Viable Hospital Podiatry Section.
Hosp. Pod. Review, Vol. 1, Fall issue, 1973.

Marlette, J. J.: Podiatry and Medicine: Partners in Health Care.
Pa. Med. 73:37, 1971.

Mercado, O. A.: Surgical Privileges for Podiatrist.
Hosp. Podiatry Review Vol. 1, Fall Issue, 1973.

Podell, R. N.: Issues in the Organization of Medical Care,
A. Illustrative Case Study—Podiatry in the United States.
N. Engl. J. Med. 284-18, Mar. 1971.

Porterfield, J. D.: The Podiatrist in the Hospital.
J.A.P.A. Vol. 60, Dec. 1970.

Puch, H. L.: Podiatry—A Boon Not a Boondoggle.
Virginia Med. Monthly, 96, Oct. 19, 1968.

Rakow, Robert B.: Out Patient Surgery in a Medical Center.
J.A.P.A. Vol. 59, Mar. 1969.

Sharp. J. T.: Podiatry Service in a Suburban Hospital.
Pa. Med. 75: Oct. 72.

Sokoloff, T.: Podiatrists' Responsibility in Patient Care.
J.A.P.A. 62: 356, 1972.

Subotnick, Steven I.: The Podiatric History and Physical.
J.A.P.A. Vol. 63, No. 10, 1973.

Whittaker, D.: Podiatry in the Veterans Administration.
J.A.P.A. Vol. 0, Mar. 1969.